2-4-13

Rick —

Welcome neighbor!

Enjoy the book — Quick Fit

to stay fit!

Best wyshes

Rick

WHAT PEOPLE SAY ABOUT QUICK FIT

I hate to do something just for exercise, but I can sneak Quick Fit in. At noontime, I walk to the grocery store or to the library. At night, I do the rest while I'm watching TV. I never have to pay attention to the fact that I'm exercising.

—PAULINE

Before Quick Fit, I had aches and pains and fatigue that I thought were just part of getting older. But now all my "growing older" symptoms have melted away. At age fifty-one, I have the energy level and stamina of a woman in her late twenties. Quick Fit turned out to be the fountain of youth for me.

—NANCY

Sometimes if I need a boost in the middle of my workday, I close my office door and do Quick Fit. This pushes the Reset button for me.

—ANTHONY

I think this system is terrific! Knowing that it's only fifteen minutes makes it so easy to get started—and to fit it into my schedule.

—JANINE

Quick Fit supplements the other exercise I do (biking, yoga, weights). It "covers" me on days when I can't squeeze in a more ambitious workout.

—CHUCK

Quick Fit appeals on many levels. I like the fact that it's fifteen minutes a day. I like that most of the time is walking, because that's familiar and I know it delivers results. I like that it's simple. You don't have to keep looking at diagrams to see if you're doing something right.

—BOB

I had let migraines and neck problems and time constraints render me inactive, even when I felt well enough to exercise. Because I didn't have time to drive to my exercise class and back, I did nothing. I felt that I was at the mercy of my own weak resolve. But Quick Fit is manageable and it's realistic time-wise.

—ROWSHANA

What makes Quick Fit work for me is not having to go to a special place or to change my clothes. There's no special equipment other than the weights. I'm never so busy that I can't take fifteen minutes.

—CLARE

Quick Fit can be sandwiched in with other activities. The other day I was making dinner and I put the potatoes on to boil. I said, "Heck, I'll just march for ten minutes." Then it was, "Well, I've got that done, so I'll do the abs." Before my potatoes were finished cooking, I had completed the whole workout.

—ANNE

The routine is so simple that I've finally overcome the barriers that kept me from exercise. I feel proud of myself.

—KIRSTEN

I have post-polio weakness in my right leg and rheumatoid arthritis affecting joints throughout my body. I might have started a big elaborate program, but I never would have continued. Quick Fit is fast and easy, and also within my physical capabilities, so it's something I can do.

—TONI

QUICK
FIT

QUICK FIT

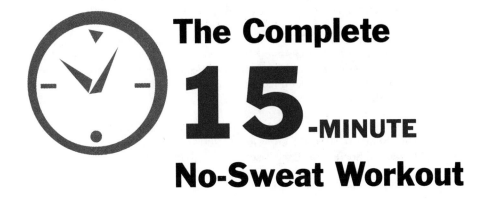

The Complete
15-MINUTE
No-Sweat Workout

Richard R. Bradley III

with Sarah Wernick

ATRIA BOOKS

New York   London   Toronto   Sydney

ATRIA BOOKS

1230 Avenue of the Americas
New York, NY 10020

The data on page 25 showing calories burned and reduction in risk of death,
were adapted with permission from *LifeFit: An Effective Excercise Program for
Optimal Health and a Longer Life,* by Ralph S. Paffenbarger, Jr., M.D. and Eric
Olsen (Human Kinetics, 1996), page 25.

The quotation from Steven N. Blair, P.E.D. on page 33 appeared in the January
1999 issue of *Nutrition Action Healthletter.* Copyright © 1999 CSPI. Reprinted
with permission from *Nutrition Action Healthletter,* Center for Science in the
Public Interest, 1875 Connecticut Ave., N.W., Suite 300, Washington DC 20009-
5728. $24.00 for 10 issues.

The PAR-Q test on page 87 is from the Physical Activity Readiness
Questionnaire (PAR-Q), copyright © 2002. Reprinted with permission from the
Canadian Society for Excercise Physiology. *http://www.csep.ca/forms.asp*

ISBN: 0-7434-7102-4

First Atria Books hardcover edition January 2004

10   9   8   7   6   5   4   3   2   1

ATRIA BOOKS is a trademark of Simon & Schuster, Inc.

Manufactured in the United States of America

Designed by Jaime Putorti

For information regarding special discounts for bulk purchases,
please contact Simon & Schuster Special Sales at 1-800-456-6798
or business@simonandschuster.com

CONTENTS

ACKNOWLEDGMENTS

I'm truly blessed that so many wonderful people have supported me in this endeavor. I thank God for all of them.

My approach to physical activity—both personally and professionally—was shaped at the University of Maryland, where I attended college. I was inspired by Dr. George Kramer and Dr. Joe Murray, my professors and coaches. They instilled in me an appreciation for an active, healthy lifestyle, as well as the values of discipline and commitment. Participating in the university's Gymkana Troupe gave me invaluable experience in performing and speaking in front of large audiences.

For the past twenty-five years, I've directed the Fitness Center at the United States Department of Transportation. Heartfelt appreciation to my supervisors, Ron Keefer, Janet Krause, and Linda Rhoads, who have supported me 100 percent. They encouraged me to reach a broad cross-section of DOT employees, including those with disabilities. And they challenged me to motivate the unmotivated. A special thanks to Hy Levasseur, my DOT colleague for twenty-three and a half years, for all that he has taught me about life as well as fitness.

I am extremely grateful to Rita Devine, a longtime family friend, who sparked the collaboration between my fitness background and the business savvy of her daughter, Maury Devine. The result is our company: Rick's Quick Fit, LLC.

With great appreciation and enthusiasm, I would like to thank Maury Devine for her persistent guidance and direction in all phases and aspects of this business. Without her unique ability to make things happen, and the positive spirit she continually exudes, this book simply would not have been possible.

I was delighted when freelance journalist Martha Frase-Blunt decided to write an article about Quick Fit for the *Washington Post*. And I was thrilled by the strong interest the article drew from NBC's *Today* show, C-SPAN, the *Voice of America*, and Mark Fenton's PBS series *America's Walking*.

A few months after the *Washington Post* article appeared, I received a letter from Sarah Wernick, an award-winning health writer, asking me if I'd be interested in writing a book about Quick Fit. We got together, agreed to collaborate—and my adventure in publishing began. Sarah's ability to translate my words and thoughts into written text is absolutely phenomenal. Thank you so much for a fantastic experience, Sarah! With your assistance, I truly believe we can make a difference in many lives.

From the first time I met Jane Dystel, my agent, and

Miriam Goderich, her partner in Dystel & Goderich Literary Management, I knew we had a winning team. Their upbeat, positive attitude, along with their vast literary management experience, have skillfully guided this journey.

I was thrilled when Atria decided to publish this book. Their enthusiasm and great ideas contributed so much. A big thank-you to Judith Curr, the publisher, who was behind us from our very first meeting. I'm deeply grateful to Tracy Behar, our editor, for her careful comments on the manuscript and for all her wonderful support at every stage. Wendy Walker, Tracy's assistant, provided much-appreciated logistical help.

I never realized how many steps it takes to transform a manuscript into a book and to bring it to readers. How fortunate I am to have the support of Atria's extraordinary team.

I'm very grateful to all the people who worked so hard to make this book look terrific. My thanks to Paolo Pepe and Patrick Kang for designing such an attractive cover, and to David Sharp, who took the excellent cover photograph. Linda Dingler and Jaime Putorti came up with a wonderful design for the inside of the book. Joe Tessmer's fine photographs provided the basis for the illustrations. Jackie Aher's excellent drawings clarify the instructions. What a delight to work with all of them.

My thanks to John Paul Jones for shepherding the book through this process. I'm grateful to Shelly Perron for her careful review of the manuscript, and to Nancy Wolff for preparing the fine index.

ACKNOWLEDGMENTS

My goal in writing this book is to reach people who can benefit from Quick Fit. Atria's splendid marketing, publicity, and sales departments have given invaluable support. I'm very grateful to Karen Mender, deputy publisher, for overseeing these efforts with exceptional skill and enthusiasm. My thanks to Seale Ballenger and Audra Boltion for their remarkable expertise and promotional zeal; to Craig Herman and Shannon McKenna, brilliant marketers; and to Larry Norton and his wonderful sales team.

This book benefited greatly from the wisdom of experts and the experiences of people who have followed the Quick Fit program.

My appreciation for permission to quote their sage words to: Steven Blair, P.E.D., Director of Research, Cooper Institute for Aerobics Research; Harvey Lauer, President of American Sports Data, Inc.; and Ralph S. Paffenbarger, Jr., M.D., Dr. P.H., Sc.D., Professor of Epidemiology, Emeritus, Stanford University School of Medicine.

Many thanks to Nancy Solkowski and Kirsten Oldenburg, who allowed me to tell their inspiring stories, and to the men and women who agreed to test the version of Quick Fit presented in this book: Janine Adams, Bob Bittner, Anthony Buscemi, Clare Donelan, Chuck Remsberg, Anne, Joan, Pauline, and Rowshana. I benefited so much from their feedback and appreciate their willingness to share their experiences with readers. Particular thanks to test group member Dr. Tina Tessina for her insights into the emotional aspects of exercise, which were so helpful.

Three splendid writers—Anita Bartholomew, Sally Wendkos Olds, and Barbara Sofer—offered detailed comments on nearly every chapter of this book, greatly improving its clarity and tone. Eve Golden, as well as Dodi Schultz and members of Compuserve's *The Right Words* forum, contributed their wisdom about wording and fine points of grammar. Willie Lockeretz reviewed the entire manuscript, making many valuable suggestions concerning content and language. My warm thanks to all of them.

My appreciation to Michael Subelsky, who designed the exciting web site for Rick's Quick Fit, LLC: *http://www.ricks quickfit.com*. Come have a look!

I'm deeply grateful for the constant support and encouragement of my close friends: Robert Caldwell, Joe Watts, Ley Mills, Fred Altiere, Lou Boland Jr., Charles Minear, Don Bordine, Peter Vendt, and Tony Buscemi.

Members of my family, the most important people in my life, have done so much to encourage me. My sisters—Robin, Sharon, and Claire—have supported me throughout my career. My sister-in-law, Jackie Gargus, always provided lots of enthusiasm in support of this project. My parents, Dick and Pat Bradley, who both started Quick Fit while I was writing this book, are an inspiration. Their success with this program proves that it's never too late to get fit. My son, Ryan, who's a business graduate of Loyola College in Baltimore, Maryland, not only keeps me on my toes as a tennis player, but also comes up with brilliant ideas for selling books.

ACKNOWLEDGMENTS

My wife, Judy, my greatest inspiration, has been by my side throughout the entire process of writing this book. Her constant support and her willingness to give her time, effort, and energy have been a tremendous encouragement to me. Judy, you're terrific—thanks, baby!

AN IMPORTANT MESSAGE FOR READERS

Quick Fit is a program of moderate-intensity physical activity, intended for healthy adults who are currently sedentary. But a published fitness program can't possibly meet the particular needs of every individual. Nor is this book intended to provide medical advice. Some exercises may be inappropriate for people with certain physical limitations.

If you are under treatment for any condition, or if you have questions or concerns, please consult a qualified professional who can examine you and provide appropriate guidance.

The authors specifically disclaim all responsibility for any liability, loss, or risk, personal or otherwise, that is incurred as a consequence, directly or indirectly, of the use and application of any components of this exercise program.

FITNESS SHOULD BE SIMPLE

I'm sedentary by nature. I walk my dog, but it's not aerobic activity. I'd like to get myself moving without holding a leash.

　　　　　　　　　　—JANINE

I exercised regularly for about ten years. Then I accepted a promotion. Previously, I was responsible for ten people; now I'm responsible for 1,500 people. I start work earlier in the morning and finish later at night. My fitness routine has been disrupted, and I want to reestablish it.

　　　　　　　　　　—ANTHONY

Since my mother's death a few years ago and my husband's cancer diagnosis last year, I've gained a lot of weight. My diet is pretty good, but I have trouble exercising enough to burn extra calories. I'm hoping to learn a routine I can do daily, one that's simple and quick enough so that I remain motivated.

—TINA

Do you wish you were fitter and healthier? You know you should exercise—but it's just not happening. There's no time, and you don't really enjoy it, so you can't get started. Maybe you're held back by extra pounds, bad knees, or another physical problem that limits your mobility. Or perhaps you're facing one of those life challenges—unemployment, a crisis with a teenager, serious illness—that makes even eating and sleeping difficult. So exercise has gone out the window.

Believe me, I understand. I've been in the fitness business for nearly thirty years. Over the decades I've worked with kids, frail senior citizens, new moms, executives who clock sixteen-hour days, professional athletes—you name it. I know how tough it can be to make exercise a regular part of your life. That's why I designed Quick Fit, and that's why I wrote this book.

Quick Fit is a complete workout, but all it takes is fifteen minutes a day. And I really mean fifteen minutes. This is no-sweat exercise. You don't need another five minutes to change clothes before you start, even if you're wearing dress-for-success business attire. You don't have to allow ten minutes to shower and get dressed afterward. Quick Fit can be done at home, at work, or anywhere your travels take you. The program is simple and realistic; it's safe—and it's efficient.

Janine, Anthony, and Tina aren't sedentary anymore. They've become consistent about exercise. You read what they said before they tried Quick Fit. Here's what they reported less than two weeks later:

> *I started the exercises and have done them seven out of the last ten days. This is huge progress for me. I think the program is terrific!*
>
> *—JANINE*

> *After laying off exercise for a month, it feels good to get back. I do Quick Fit first thing in the morning, and it starts the day with a real boost.*
>
> *—ANTHONY*

> *On the first day, I began with the first exercise, thinking I'd do as much as I could. I wound up going all the way to the end. The ease of the whole thing—the small amount of time, not needing to go anywhere or to wear special clothing—makes it work for me.*
>
> *—TINA*

Janine, Anthony, and Tina were part of a group that tested the program in this book. I want you to know something that makes me particularly excited about their success: They started Quick Fit in mid-December, right between Thanksgiving and Christmas. Imagine learning a new exercise program—and finding the time to do it—during that hectic period. What an accomplishment! But Quick Fit is so simple and convenient that they didn't want to wait—and they didn't have to. I promise: This program will get *you* moving, too.

THE STORY OF QUICK FIT

I'm one of those people who actually prefers running to sitting. My mother tells me I was born moving. (She also tells me, "Slow down!") Because I enjoy physical activity so much, I've always coaxed others to join me. I take it as a personal challenge to convince anyone who's sedentary—even people who say they hate exercise—to give it a try. I've converted thousands.

In college, at the University of Maryland, I joined the Gymkana Troupe, an exhibitional gymnastics team. Unlike other collegiate gymnastic teams, we didn't compete. Our purpose was to have a great time and to promote healthy drug-free living through our performances in schools and community centers. I loved it! I know this sounds crazy if you've never been a gymnast, but even now, when I'm past fifty, I still do handstands on the parallel bars in my basement. My wife, Judy, shakes her head when she watches me turn upside down. "Rick," she says, "no wonder your hair is still red."

During my freshman year in college, I heard about a field called industrial fitness. American businesses, inspired by the Japanese, were incorporating exercise into the workplace. They had learned that when you boost fitness, you boost productivity. I knew this was the perfect career for me; I loved the idea of working with companies to help their employees get fit. I majored in physical education and exercise physiology, and graduated from the University of Maryland with honors in 1975. The following year I received national certification in occupational health from the YMCA.

My first job out of college was as program director for Health and Fitness at the local YMCA. Three years later, I joined the Occupational Health and Fitness Program at the United States Department of Transportation (DOT)—and I've been there ever since.

Throughout my long and happy affiliation with DOT, I've also consulted on fitness. In the early 1980s I was flexibility coach for the Washington Redskins football team under their legendary coach Joe Gibbs. I started my own company, Creative Stress Management, in 1983. Through this business I've conducted seminars on health and fitness for hundreds of companies, schools, churches, community centers, and other organizations.

The Best Program in the World

Back in the 1970s and 1980s, the fitness regimens I recommended required forty-five minutes a day: thirty minutes of aerobics, ten minutes of strength training, and five minutes of stretches. I thought this was the best program in the world. Of course, by the time someone showered and changed clothes, the whole routine took more than an hour. As far as I was concerned, that seemed about right. But people kept telling me: "I don't have time for this." Or they'd do it for a while, then begin to skip exercise sessions, and finally quit.

It wasn't just average folks who had trouble sticking with the workouts I designed. When I worked for the Washington Redskins, I came up with a stretching program for the team. I explained to these massive guys how much it would help them if they stretched: "Your muscles contract all the time. Here's a routine that will stretch them out again. It will improve your performance and reduce the risk of injury. All it takes is forty-five minutes a day."

You know what they said? "Fat chance."

Over the years, I've watched people start many other exercise programs. Members of the DOT Fitness Center often bring in the latest books to ask me what I think. You've seen these books. Some of them feature "before" pictures, showing flabby men and women with dull skin and stringy hair. In the "after" pictures, they're not only trim and muscular, they've also got shiny skin and attractive hairdos. Isn't that amazing?

But what I want to know is: Where are the *"after* after*"* pictures? Most of these programs are demanding, with lengthy, shirt-drenching workouts. I recently saw a book that called for a *minimum* of five thirty-minute aerobic workouts per week, preferably involving strenuous activities like jogging or climbing stairs. You could climb a skyscraper in thirty minutes. Do you know anyone who does that five days a week?

I'm not knocking these books. People who consistently follow their recommendations get great results. If you can keep up an hour-plus per-day commitment to strenuous exercise, more power to you. But in my experience—and survey findings back this up—most people simply can't; they quit in a couple of weeks. Sometimes they last a few months, but then they become increasingly inconsistent and finally stop altogether. Worst of all, they feel bad about themselves and discouraged about exercise.

Years ago, I'd shrug it off when people quit an exercise program, whether it was one of my lengthy routines or someone else's. I'd think, okay, that's their choice. I didn't yet understand a very important principle: If people won't follow an exercise program, it's *not* the best program in the world.

How Much Exercise Do We Really Need?

In the 1970s, when I studied exercise physiology at the University of Maryland, experts believed that the only way to get any beneficial results was to work out vigorously for at least twenty minutes. But subsequent studies showed that moderate exercise was just as effective. Moreover, less vigorous exercise caused fewer injuries.

For example, you get about the same health benefit—and burn about the same number of calories—whether you walk one mile or run the same distance. Of course, you can complete that mile more quickly if you run. But walking is safer. You're less likely to sprain an ankle or hurt your knees or other vulnerable joints.

Another advance was the discovery that short exercise sessions can make a real difference. These findings were summarized in the 1996 *Surgeon General's Report on Physical Activity and Health*. I read the report with great interest. One statement jumped out at me:

> *People who are usually inactive can improve their health and well-being by becoming even moderately active on a regular basis.*

In other words:

- Even if you've been sedentary, it's never too late to begin exercising.
- Exercise need not be strenuous to improve health and well-being.
- What's important is making exercise a regular part of your life.

By then, my own thinking had evolved considerably. I understood—especially after I got married and my son, Ryan, was born—that finding time really was tough for people who are working and dealing with family responsibilities, and who don't necessarily love physical activity the way I do. They don't want to wake up an hour early so they can do forty-five minutes of exercise, then shower and dress; nor do they want to spend that much time at the end of a busy day, when they're tired and hungry for dinner. Who could blame them?

Finally, I realized: *The best exercise program in the world is one that people will do consistently.* Such a program must be simple, convenient, and realistic; it must fit into people's lives. Was it possible, I wondered, to develop an exercise routine that would take just fifteen minutes, yet provide a meaningful workout? I decided to give it a shot.

Packing a Complete Workout into Fifteen Minutes

The task was challenging. My workout had to cover the key components of exercise—aerobic activity, strength training, and stretches for flexibility—in just a quarter of an hour. Every move would have to deliver multiple benefits. But a program for people who are reluctant to exercise would also need to be simple to learn and easy to do.

I decided that ten minutes out of the fifteen would be devoted to a brisk walk—aerobic exercise to condition the heart and lungs. Walking is the perfect aerobic activity: It can be done anytime and anyplace. No equipment is required; no instructions are needed.

That left five minutes for strength and flexibility. Since walking strengthens the leg muscles, I focused on the midsection and upper body. Everyone wants toned abdominal muscles, so I added one minute of abdominal crunches. There are many ways to perform ab exercises; I picked a version that also strengthens the neck muscles. Four minutes remained.

I selected three strengthening exercises for the upper body that would require about one minute each. Together, they address muscles in the back, shoulders, chest, upper arms, forearms, and wrists. And because these exercises move the arms through their full range of motion, they improve flexibility, too.

The clock was ticking! Just one minute for stretching. I picked one stretch for the upper body and one for the lower body. Thirty seconds each. The upper body stretch includes a strengthening component for the shoulders, a little bonus. The lower body stretch is pure relaxation—the perfect way to end a workout.

I called this program Quick Fit. Fifteen minutes from start to finish. Now *that's* quick, and you get fit!

> *Inch by inch,*
> *fitness is a cinch.*
> *Yard by yard*
> *makes it hard.*

Quick Fit Catches On

I introduced Quick Fit at the Department of Transportation Fitness Center in 1998. Everyone who tried the program loved it. They told their friends and coworkers. More people came to the Fitness Center than ever before.

That wasn't enough for me. I went around the building, recruiting. I'd arrive at one of the office suites and ask the receptionist, "Did anyone here call me to learn about Quick Fit?" The receptionist would go around to the cubicles and ask, "Who wanted to hear about Quick Fit?" That made everyone curious. Note that I didn't say anyone had actually called, because the truth was, no one had. But inevitably, a crowd would gather in the reception area. People would be asking, "What's Quick Fit?" So I'd say, "Well, as long as you're here, let me tell you about it . . ."

Pretty soon, hundreds of DOT employees were doing Quick Fit. The program also was a hit with the thousands of people who've attended the wellness seminars I offer through my consulting company, Creative Stress Management.

A journalist who heard about Quick Fit, Martha Frase-Blunt, decided to write an article about it for the *Washington Post*. She visited DOT, interviewed me, and spoke to people there who were doing the program.

The article was published on August 21, 2001. Hours after the paper hit the newsstands, NBC's *Today* show called. The next day they sent a camera crew to the Fitness Center at DOT and I was on the air. What a thrill!

Though I was delighted by the interest in Quick Fit, the beginning of the article made me a little uncomfortable. Here's what it said:

It's 10 A.M. in the lobby of the U.S. Department of Transportation's vast headquarters in L'Enfant Plaza and Rick Bradley has just spotted his day's first mark. The man—harried, 40-ish, with a thick waist, tired eyes and a slightly stunned expression—gets on the elevator, and Bradley follows. "Hey," he greets the unsuspecting man as the doors slide shut.

I expressed my concern to my wife: "It sounds as if I pursue people."

"Wait a minute," Judy said. "Isn't that exactly what you do?"

I have to admit it: I'm not shy about approaching out-of-shape colleagues at the Department of Transportation. Now I'm reaching out to everyone with a book about Quick Fit. I've adapted the exercises so you can do them anywhere, without expensive equipment. If you're sedentary and wish you were at a different level of fitness, I want to tell you what I told that guy in the elevator:

You don't need a whole new lifestyle to change your life dramatically. Just a little bit of exercise can make a difference.

WHAT REGULAR EXERCISE CAN DO FOR YOU

No pill can match the health benefits of exercise. Regular physical activity cuts the risk of heart disease and stroke, counters excess weight and diabetes, and protects against certain forms of cancer. What's more, people who exercise are happier and more productive.

Nevertheless, many Americans have taken the call to fitness lying down. A recent government survey asked adults if they exercise in their leisure time. Any physical activity—even a ten-minute walk—qualified for a "yes." But an astonishing 38 percent said "no."

Why don't more people exercise? The number one reason: Lack of time.

Can Fifteen Minutes Really Make a Difference?

You may have heard that you must work out for at least thirty minutes to experience any benefit. Or you may think that physical activity doesn't count unless your heart pounds and your clothes are soaked with sweat.

Not so! Exercise, like money in the bank, is cumulative. It all adds up.

People ask me: "Can Quick Fit provide all the beneficial effects of exercise programs that call for longer and more strenuous workouts?" I tell them: "It depends on whether you'll actually do those workouts."

Think of the bank again. If you deposit $15 a week, your

balance won't be as high as if you deposit $30 a week. But a *consistent* $15 per week beats an irregular $30 every month or so—and it's a whole lot better than nothing. That's true for exercise, too.

A woman raised her hand at one of my seminars. She said, "Rick, I walk on the treadmill for half an hour five times a week. After three of those sessions I add a twenty-minute workout with weights. And I have a five-minute stretching routine that I do after each workout." Some of the other people in the audience looked ready to collapse, just from listening to her. She asked, "Should I drop this and do Quick Fit instead?"

"No—don't stop! What you're doing is great," I told her. "But you might want to try Quick Fit on those two days when you don't exercise, or when you can't manage your usual program."

Many people who normally follow more demanding exercise routines turn to Quick Fit when time is tight. For example, Chuck says:

Yesterday I had about half an hour before an appointment. Quick Fit fit perfectly into that opening, which I probably would have frittered away otherwise.

Unfortunately, the folks who need to exercise the most can't (or won't) work out thirty-plus minutes a day, month after month, year after year. They resolve to exercise on January 1; they buy a treadmill on the cable TV shopping channel. Then a couple of months later, they've quit and they're using the treadmill as a coatrack. But lifelong fitness requires consistency.

People who won't do any other exercise are willing to try Quick Fit. It allows them to ease into fitness with minimal risk of injury. Once they start, nearly all of them stick with it, because it's so easy—and because it makes them feel so good.

Small Efforts, Big Payoffs

Results start with the very first workout. I'm not promising that you'll be transformed, in just fifteen minutes, into someone your best friend wouldn't recognize. But when you're done, you'll definitely feel energized. You'll probably have a smile on your face, too, because physical activity is a natural mood booster. And if you've been plagued by guilt because you can't get yourself to exercise, imagine the relief—and pride—when you finally begin.

Over time, other benefits develop. Your heart and lungs become stronger, so you have more energy and stamina. You might not notice this if the rest of your life is sedentary. But one of these days you'll play tennis or take a long walk, or you'll shop and lug heavy bags back from the store—and suddenly you'll realize that this exertion is much easier than it would have been before Quick Fit.

Once you're stronger and fitter, physical activity won't seem like such a chore. In fact, it might actually be fun. For many people, Quick Fit is a bridge to a more active, healthier lifestyle.

What About Weight Loss?

People often ask me if Quick Fit will help them lose weight. The answer is yes—but this isn't a weight-loss program. One Quick Fit session burns approximately fifty to seventy-five extra calories per day. Obviously, that's not as much as you'd burn if you were in training for the Olympics. But it sure beats a day at the computer followed by an evening on the sofa.

If you add a daily Quick Fit workout to whatever other exercise you're doing (if any)—and you don't alter your diet or anything else in your life—you'd lose about five pounds in a year. If you lost five pounds a year starting at age forty-five, you'd be down twenty-five pounds by the time you hit your half-century birthday.

What often happens, though, is that when people who've been sedentary start exercising consistently with Quick Fit, they begin to make other changes in their lives. And that's when the weight really comes off. What's more, stronger abdominal muscles flatten their midsections and help them stand taller. Those changes make them look trimmer, too.

> *To lose weight,*
> *move a little more;*
> *eat a little less.*

Nancy lost eighty-five pounds, and it all began with Quick Fit. When she joined the DOT Fitness Center four years ago, her energy level was down and her weight was up. She didn't think she had time for exercise, so I started her on Quick Fit. She became a regular at the Fitness Center.

A few months after she joined, Nancy attended one of the nutrition seminars we offer from time to time. She decided to cut back on the fat in her diet, and to eat more fruits and vegetables. She also added more exercises to her workout. A year later, she was eighty-five pounds lighter—and she's kept the weight off ever since. Says Nancy:

> *I don't look as if I've lost eighty-five pounds; I look completely different. I used to shop from catalogs for large-size women; now I can shop at Victoria's Secret. A good friend who hadn't seen me for a while walked right past me at a conference. I called her name. She stopped, looked at me, and said, "I recognize the voice, but I can't seem to place you." I told her, "It's Nancy." She was amazed. She kept saying, "I can't believe it—I just can't believe it!"*

WHAT'S IN THE BOOK?

Quick Fit is so simple, I could show you the moves in just a few minutes. But there's more to developing a lifelong fitness habit than learning the exercises. You must be motivated. You need to understand what's been holding you back, so you can figure out how to overcome the obstacles that have tripped you up in the past. Once you've started and have been exercising for a while, it's helpful to think about how you'll keep up your good work. That's what this book is all about.

If you're impatient to begin, you don't have to read the whole book first. Turn to page 101 for Quick Start.

Most people know that exercise is good for them. But they're amazed when they find out just how many benefits they can expect from fitness, even if they're spending only fifteen minutes a day. Chapter 2 explains why you need to get moving and tells you about some of the latest research findings on exercise.

When I give seminars, I always ask people to raise their hands if they exercise regularly. Usually, very few hands go up. Then I ask: Why not? Occasionally, the problem is an injury or a difficult personal situation that takes priority over everything else. But mostly I simply hear excuses. In Chapter 3 I'll list the most common problems—and explain how to get past them. I'll also explain how exercise can actually help when life pitches you a curve.

Quick Fit takes very little time from your day. But it does require a commitment. I'll talk about that in Chapter 4, suggesting ways you can commit to getting fit.

No one should start an exercise program without checking to see if they need medical clearance. In Chapter 5, I'll give you a simple test to see if you must discuss this program with your doctor before you begin; you can adapt the exercises to most personal limitations. This chapter prepares you to begin the program, with information about everything from setting up a small workout space to making sure your shoes fit properly.

After you're pumped and prepared, it's time to learn Quick Fit's simple moves. Chapter 6 walks you through the exercises, step by step.

Developing an exercise habit is much easier if you make it fun. In Chapter 7, I'll give you many ideas, as well as suggestions for staying motivated.

You can continue doing Quick Fit forever. But many sedentary people who follow the program are astonished to discover that they actually enjoy physical activity. They love their trimmer, tighter bodies; they relish their improved energy. Suddenly, fifteen minutes isn't enough. That's great news, because you gain even more benefits if you expand the Quick Fit workout. I'll explain how to do that—without overdoing and burning out—in Chapter 8.

Any questions? In Chapter 9 I'll answer the ones I hear most often when I talk to people about Quick Fit.

Consistency is the name of the game with fitness exercise. If you can stay consistent with Quick Fit for four months, you've established a habit—and you'll also see results. Chapter 10 gives you a month-by-month preview of those important first months.

QUICK FIT

I know you want to get fit, because you picked up this book. Quick Fit is easy, realistic, and convenient. Finally, there's an exercise program you can do for life.

WHY YOU NEED TO GET MOVING

During the work-life wellness seminars I present for businesses and other organizations around the country, I meet many brilliant and highly successful executives. They've devoted a lot of time to their fiscal fitness, but in the process, they've neglected their physical fitness. I tell them:

You're spending your health to gain your wealth. But later on, you're going to have to spend that wealth to regain your health.

Fitness is the single factor that best predicts how long you will live. You probably realize that exercise is good for your heart. But did you know that physical activity protects against cancer, too? This chapter describes all the benefits you can expect if you do Quick Fit every day—and there are many more than you might imagine. Being fit isn't just about the *quantity* of life; it's about the *quality* of life. Active people aren't just healthier, they're happier, too.

When you're already active, it's exciting to read about the gains you get from exercise. When you're sedentary, you may wonder if you've missed the boat. Here's some great news: Quick Fit helps everyone—but those who benefit the most are the people who are completely inactive now. What's more, it's *never* too late to get started!

HOW MUCH EXERCISE MAKES A DIFFERENCE?

Fifteen minutes of daily physical activity makes a significant difference for your health. What? Only fifteen minutes?

I know you've read that we need a lot more than that. In 2002, the National Academies' Institute of Medicine announced that to maintain optimal cardiovascular health, Americans should spend a total of at least one hour each day in moderately intense physical activity. One hour! You could hear people groaning all across America. That's double the daily minimum of thirty minutes recommended in the 1996 *Surgeon General's Report on Physical Activity and Health*. And as the surgeon general's report acknowledged, more than 60 percent of Americans don't do even that much.

Fortunately, exercise is not an all-or-nothing proposition. An hour would be outstanding; thirty minutes would be excellent. But research shows that even a smaller amount of exercise is meaningful.

Evidence from the College Alumni Health Study

For every hour a person exercises, he or she gets back that hour plus an extra hour of life.
—DR. RALPH PAFFENBARGER, FOUNDER OF THE COLLEGE ALUMNI HEALTH STUDY

Much of what we know about the long-term benefits of exercise comes from several major studies that have followed thousands of people for decades. One of the most ambitious is the College Alumni Health Study. Since 1960, this study has tracked the health and lifestyles of more than 40,000 men and women who attended Harvard and the University of Pennsylvania between 1916 and 1950. The surviving participants now range in age from 70 to over 100.

Why focus on Harvard and Penn? Not because of their Ivy League status, but because these two colleges have given entering freshmen thorough physical examinations since the early 1900s—and they kept all the records. Researchers could contact former students and match their current health information with medical records from their teen years.

To update information about participants, the College Alumni Health Study regularly mails them questionnaires. One focus is physical activity. How many blocks do they walk each day? How many stairs do they climb? Do they play any sports? Researchers convert the answers into the approximate number of calories burned. For example, climbing and descending five flights of stairs is rated at 40 calories; walking one mile is rated at 100 calories.

The study has found significant health benefits in those who burn a total of just 500 to 1,000 calories per week in physical activity. If you do Quick Fit every day, you'd burn about 500 calories in a week. That's how we know that fifteen minutes of exercise can make a meaningful difference.

A Dose of Exercise

With most medication, the more you take (up to a point), the greater the benefit you can expect. For example, if you have a headache, one pain pill might take the edge off your discomfort, while two will relieve it entirely. This is called a dose-response relationship. Exercise works the same way: The more you do (up to a point), the more benefit you can expect.

Have a look at the numbers on the next page, from the College Alumni Health Study. The lifestyle change that gives the biggest bang for the buck is going from nothing to 500 calories. In other words, if you're completely sedentary, it really pays to start Quick Fit! Interestingly, with exercise, as with nearly everything else, you can get too much of a good thing: Those who exercised the most were not the ones who lived longest.

Calories Burned per Week in Exercise	Reduction in Risk of Death
0	0%
500–1000	27%
1,000–1,500	29%
1,500–2,000	36%
2,000–2,500	43%
2,500–3,000	26%
3,000–3,500	19%

Source: *LifeFit: An Effective Exercise Program for Optimal Health and a Longer Life*, by Ralph S. Paffenbarger Jr., M.D., and Eric Olsen (Human Kinetics, 1996), page 25.

As you can see, the greatest health benefits were enjoyed by those who burn about 2,000 calories per week. What does it take to burn 2,000 calories? A brisk one-hour walk every day would do it. Findings like these explain why the National Academies' Institute of Medicine would like all of us to get an hour of daily exercise. If you can achieve that goal, terrific! But if you can't, don't let that discourage you from doing less.

With exercise, *anything* is much better than *nothing*.

BEHIND THE MAGIC OF PHYSICAL ACTIVITY

Other major studies confirm that fitness is the key to longevity. For example, the Cooper Institute for Aerobics

Research has compiled records and follow-up data from more than 32,000 men and women who have undergone comprehensive health examinations at the Institute's clinic in Dallas, Texas. All participants were extensively questioned about their medical history and smoking habits. To determine if they were overweight, they were weighed and measured for height. And everyone took a treadmill test to rate their level of fitness. Those who could manage only a slow walk scored low; those fit enough to run with the treadmill on an incline scored high.

When the investigators looked at follow-up data, they discovered that the single most powerful predictor of mortality was the treadmill test result. In other words: Fitness. Those in the lowest fitness category had *double* the death rate of those with medium or high fitness levels. Except for smoking, no other risk factor came close.

Why does physical activity make such a big difference? Let me tell you what happens when someone clicks off the TV, hauls himself out of the recliner, and goes out for a brisk walk. All the systems of the body leap into action.

- Muscles in the feet, legs, torso, back, shoulders, arms, and hands contract and relax, moving the body along.
- The heart and all the blood vessels work harder to move blood through the body. That's because active muscles need extra oxygen and nutrients. Also, as they burn fuel, muscles create waste that must be carried away via the bloodstream.

- The lungs process more air, bringing in oxygen and getting rid of carbon dioxide.
- The central nervous system goes on alert, helping the body stay coordinated and balanced.
- The skeleton is stimulated to produce bone tissue.
- The brain takes on additional administrative chores, making sure that the body responds properly to the increased demands of physical activity.
- Beneficial biochemical changes occur throughout the body to support all these efforts.

Quick Fit mobilizes all of these systems. Over time, the systems adapt to the increased demand: Either they develop the capacity to work harder, or they learn to work more efficiently. In the process, all the systems improve.

EXERCISE FIGHTS THE LEADING CAUSES OF EARLY DEATH

Every year, the National Center for Health Statistics publishes the ten leading causes of death in the United States. When I read that list, I feel the same way that I do when I see the FBI's "Most Wanted" poster in the post office: I want to fight those bad guys!

Did you know that the American Heart Association now includes a sedentary lifestyle as a major risk factor for heart attacks and stroke? Heart disease is the number one killer;

stroke is number three. Think about that: Lack of exercise is right up there with high cholesterol, high blood pressure, smoking, obesity, and diabetes. Furthermore, heart disease and stroke aren't the only major killers to which inactivity contributes. Lack of exercise is a risk factor for three more of the top ten: cancer, diabetes, and chronic lower respiratory disease.

Heart Disease

As we get older, there's a natural reduction in our cardiac power. Even if we stay fit, the heart simply can't beat as fast as it could in our younger years. However, most of us lose a lot more cardiac power and cardiac health from lifestyle habits—including smoking, overeating, and inactivity—than from aging.

In the College Alumni Health Study, researchers began to see the difference when the participants reached age fifty. Those who were physically active reduced their risk of death from heart attacks and strokes by about 35 percent compared to the most sedentary alumni in the study.

Regular physical activity protects the cardiovascular system by tackling the conditions that lead to heart disease:

Arterial Sclerosis

Arteries are blood vessels, the branching tubes that carry blood from the heart to the cells and organs of the body. The tissue that lines the arteries is supposed to be smooth. But sometimes the lining becomes inflamed and clogged with debris, a condition called arterial sclerosis. This damage prevents blood from flowing freely, which can cause heart attacks, strokes, and claudication (cramping pain in the legs or arms).

Though the health of our arteries is partly determined by our genes, lifestyle choices—whether we eat well, exercise, and refrain from smoking—play a major role too. We can't choose our parents, but we can decide how we live.

High Cholesterol

Cholesterol is a waxy substance that our body needs to build strong cell membranes. When too much cholesterol circulates in the blood, the excess may be deposited in the arteries, causing blockages. But cholesterol comes in different forms. The dangerous kind is low-density lipoprotein (LDL). There's also a healthy form called high-density lipoprotein (HDL), which protects the arteries by removing cholesterol deposits.

Some of the cholesterol in our blood comes from eating animal products such as meat, eggs, butter, and cheese. Cutting back on those foods may lower cholesterol levels, but not necessarily. That's because cholesterol is also manufactured by the liver. But we can improve our cholesterol numbers with physical activity. Exercise reduces LDL (the bad cholesterol) in our blood, and increases HDL (the good cholesterol). This is one of the ways that physical activity helps cut the risk of heart attacks and stroke.

High Blood Pressure

Pressure is created in the arteries when your heart pumps blood. Healthy arteries stretch to compensate. If they don't stretch properly, or if the heart pumps too hard, blood pressure will be elevated.

High blood pressure is dangerous—and not only for your heart. Among the possible consequences:

- The heart is forced to pump harder, which can weaken or damage it.
- Blood vessels throughout the body may be weakened by excess pressure; they may even break, causing internal bleeding.
- The brain is vulnerable to a stroke if a blood vessel breaks under pressure.
- Blindness can result if blood vessels in the eye rupture because of high blood pressure.
- Kidney damage can occur because blood vessels become less able to work with the kidneys to filter blood.

High blood pressure places a strain on your entire body. One in four Americans—and one in three African-Americans—has high blood pressure (also called hypertension), according to the American Heart Association. Many of them don't know it, because the condition doesn't cause symptoms at first—that's why it's sometimes called "the silent killer."

If high blood pressure runs in your family, you're at

above-average risk. However, you can improve your odds by adopting healthy habits. Regular exercise helps prevent high blood pressure and can even bring it under control after it develops. Physical activity widens the arteries, allowing blood to move more easily. It also conditions the heart, helping it to pump more efficiently with less strain.

Cancer

Many people are surprised to hear that exercise helps protect against cancer, the second leading cause of death in the United States. But it does. In the College Alumni Health Study, those who were physically active had a cancer risk nearly one-third lower than those who were sedentary. Other investigations have shown that physical activity cuts the odds of getting breast cancer, prostate cancer, colon cancer, and lung cancer, among others. What's the connection?

Cancer is triggered by a variety of factors, including exposure to toxins in the environment, cigarette smoking, and certain viruses. Exercise fights back by—

- Boosting the immune system, which is the body's defense against cancer as well as other diseases. The immune system counters the effects of carcinogens and destroys abnormal cells before they spread.
- Helping prevent obesity, which is connected to many cancers, including cancer of the breast, colon, and prostate. The reasons for this connection are not fully understood,

but experts believe that estrogen and other hormones secreted by fat tissue may stimulate cancerous growth.

- Triggering deeper, more rapid breathing, which helps clear toxins from the lungs.
- Stimulating the digestive tract, thereby moving wastes—which include carcinogens—out of the body. The less time these substances spend in contact with the lining of the colon, the less likely they are to cause colon cancer.

Diabetes

Our bodies are fueled by glucose (sugar), which is obtained from the food we eat and transported to our cells via the bloodstream. Insulin—a hormone that is secreted by the pancreas—normally helps the cells extract glucose from the blood. In diabetes, this important mechanism doesn't work properly.

In Type 1 diabetes, which usually starts in childhood, the body doesn't produce sufficient insulin. Type 2, which accounts for about 90 percent of all cases, typically begins in adulthood; the body usually produces sufficient insulin, but the cells don't use it effectively. With both forms of the disease, glucose builds up in the blood while the cells go hungry. The consequences can be devastating. Diabetes is a leading cause of heart disease, kidney failure, and blindness.

Exercise helps prevent Type 2 diabetes. In the College Alumni Health Study, the risk of getting this form of the disease was significantly lower in those who were active—and the more active they were, the more protection they enjoyed. Part of the benefit comes from the contribution that exercise makes to weight loss. But physical activity also seems to help cells respond to insulin and use glucose properly.

Regular exercise would increase average longevity by two or three years. That doesn't seem like very much, but if someone tomorrow found a magic bullet that completely cured all cancer, average longevity would increase by less than two years.
—STEVEN N. BLAIR, P.E.D., DIRECTOR OF RESEARCH, COOPER INSTITUTE FOR AEROBICS RESEARCH

THE BEST WAY TO COMBAT FAT

Americans have never been as heavy as we are now. According to the U.S. Centers for Disease Control and Prevention, three out of every five American adults weigh too much. What's piling on the pounds? It's really pretty simple: We overeat and we don't get enough exercise. In other words, blame it on a combination of supersize portions and modern labor-saving conveniences.

The Risks

I'm sure you already know that excess weight is associated with those major killers we've already discussed: heart disease, stroke, diabetes, and cancer. A study published in *Annals of Internal Medicine* in 2003 reported that people who are overweight at age forty die six to seven years earlier, on average, than those of normal weight.

People who carry extra pounds are more likely to be burdened by painful chronic conditions such as osteoarthritis, gallstones, and gout. And on top of everything else, many heavy people suffer from depression and low self-esteem.

The Solution: Exercise

If you've struggled with your weight for years, you may wonder if the situation is hopeless. It's not! Regular exercise contributes significantly to weight loss—and there's nothing better to help you maintain a healthy weight as you get older.

Losing even part of that excess weight can make a major difference for your health. Studies find that overweight people can lower their blood pressure and reduce cholesterol and blood sugar if they shed as little as 5 to 15 percent of their total body weight. In other words, someone who weighs two hundred pounds can make a significant dent in their risk of heart disease, stroke, and diabetes by dropping just 10 pounds. What's more, becoming fit can keep you healthy even if your weight doesn't change much.

Fit and Fat?

Yes, you can be fit even if you're overweight. That's right, you can increase your life span, enjoy more energy, and feel great, even if no one would mistake you for a supermodel. Data from the Cooper Institute's longevity studies show that much of the association between excess weight and early mortality can be explained by the fact that most overweight people don't get much exercise. Cooper Institute scientists have found that fat people who are physically fit actually have a lower risk of dying than unfit people of normal weight!

How Quick Fit Can Help

Quick Fit isn't a weight-loss program. But when combined with sensible eating, it can help make that valuable 5 to 15 percent difference in your weight. Kirsten joined the Department of Transportation Fitness Center shortly before her sixtieth birthday, because she wanted to gain strength and stay healthy as she aged. She says:

> *When you're overweight, you don't want to go to the gym. Rick told me about Quick Fit. The routine was so simple, he sold me. I started going to the gym every day. One thing led to another. My eating patterns weren't terrible, but I made small improvements, like adding more fruits and vegetables and cutting down on portions. In two years I've lost thirty pounds; I now wear size eight instead*

of size sixteen. My body is stronger and I feel better about myself. People tell me, "Wow, you look so good!"

FITNESS MAKES YOU FEEL BETTER NOW

Fitness doesn't just mean living longer later; it means living better right now. When you get in shape, you become a better you. You look good; you feel good; you have more energy and vitality. You're less likely to feel ill. You sleep better. Everything you do—whether it's work or play—you do more easily, without undue strain or fatigue. Not surprisingly, your mood and mental functioning are better, too.

The emotional benefits of exercise appear quickly. You will probably experience them on the very first day. In fact, exercise is so beneficial for mood that it's sometimes prescribed for people who suffer from depression. Some studies have found that aerobic activity is as potent as antidepression drugs.

What explains these emotional benefits? Some reasons are obvious. Why wouldn't we feel better if we have more energy, feel stronger, and look better?

Physical mechanisms seem to be involved as well. Exercise triggers the release of brain chemicals, called neurotransmitters, that act as mood elevators. Have you heard of "runner's high"—the euphoria that some runners experience? This reaction may be caused by the release of endorphins, opium-like chemicals that reduce pain and elevate mood. Yet another natural chemical credited with this effect is phenylethylamine. We know that phenylethylamine improves mood, and we also know that the body produces more of it during physical activity. By the way, phenylethylamine is also found in chocolate, so if you like chocolate, you should love exercise!

FITNESS IS COST-EFFECTIVE

Many leading corporations and small businesses offer exercise programs. This isn't only a matter of treating employees well. When companies crunch the numbers, they usually find that fitness programs pay for themselves. Indeed, they sometimes turn a profit. Here's what boosts the bottom line:

- Lower health care costs
- Reduced absenteeism
- Increased productivity
- Improved employee morale, which cuts turnover and draws top workers

Two award-winning—and cost-effective—programs:

Texas Instruments

Texas Instruments first brought physical activity to its work-places more than two decades ago. In 1995, TI built a $1.2 million state-of-the-art fitness facility at their Dallas head-quarters. This investment pays off—by keeping employes pro-ductive and healthy, and by making the company even more attractive to new recruits. TI also supports clubs that encourage involvement in active recreational sports, such as golf, tennis, and flag football. In recent years, with an eye to improving family health—and combating the epidemic of childhood obesity—TI has encouraged employees' kids and spouses to participate, too.

FedEx

FedEx offers a variety of programs designed to promote health and fitness, including five on-site wellness centers. Approximately 3,000 FedEx employees have joined these convenient facilities, where they can use workout equipment and attend excercise classes and nutrition seminars. Promoting a more active lifestyle is not only healthier; it has economic benefits too: Medical costs are 6 percent lower for wellness center members than for nonmember FedEx employees.

A TRUE FOUNTAIN OF YOUTH

Many of the physical changes we associate with getting older—the loss of vitality and strength, that creeping weight gain—aren't caused exclusively by age. They're also the product of inactivity. In fact, a remarkable Texas study proved that lack of exercise actually does *more* damage than aging.

Back in 1966, researchers from the Southwestern Medical School in Dallas recruited five healthy male college students for a very unusual summer job. The students underwent a complete medical and fitness evaluation, including treadmill tests—and then they spent three weeks in bed. To make sure they didn't get even the slightest amount of exercise, the students were required to use wheelchairs to visit the bathroom. After three weeks, they were retested.

This short period of inactivity produced startling declines in the strength and cardiovascular fitness of these young men. Two of the students were so weakened that they fainted during a treadmill test. Another reported that it was difficult to drive a car: The effort of pressing the brake pedal hurt his leg.

The investigation—called the Dallas Bed Rest Study— dramatically demonstrated the detrimental effects of inactivity. Because of its findings, doctors stopped advising bed rest after childbirth, surgery, and heart attacks; instead, they encouraged patients to get up and move as soon as possible.

Thirty years later, in 1996, the five former students returned to the laboratory. Not surprisingly, follow-up tests revealed that the men, now in their fifties, had lost cardiovascular capacity and strength over the previous three decades. However, they weren't as weak as they'd been in 1966 after the period of bed rest. *Just three weeks of inactivity took more of a toll than thirty years of aging.*

Later in this chapter I'll tell you more about the follow-up study. I'm sure you'll be greatly encouraged by the results.

A REAL-LIFE FITNESS TEST

How old is your body? No, I'm not asking about your age—I'm asking how fit you are for everyday activities. Take this simple test, which covers aerobic capacity, strength, balance, and flexibility. Check the box if your answer is Yes:

❑ Can you climb two flights of stairs without getting out of breath?

❑ Do you usually walk down steps without holding on to the railing?

❑ Can you rise from a low chair without using your hands?

❑ Can you put on and tie a shoe while balancing on the other foot?

❑ Can you lift a full carry-on suitcase into an overhead luggage compartment?

❑ Can you do heavy household jobs without feeling sore the next day?

❑ Can you get down on the floor and get up again without strain?

❑ When you walk with a healthy friend your own age, do you keep up?

❑ Can you reach all the parts of your body that you need to reach for dressing, grooming, and personal hygiene?

❑ Do you have the energy to enjoy life—to dance at a wedding or play volleyball at a picnic—rather than just being a spectator?

Now count the checks. That's your score. Here's what it means:

10   You're moving like a person age 20 to 39. If you're older than that, congratulations! Stay fit and you can remain youthful for many years.

7–9   Consider yourself middle-aged, fitness-wise. You're functioning like someone age 40 to 59. That's great if you're actually a senior citizen. Otherwise, you could do better if you become fitter.

4–6   Your body behaves like the body of a person age 60 to 79. This is good news if you're over 80. If not, you could turn back the clock by a decade or more if you shape up.

0–3   Your physical limitations are like those of a person age 80 or older. Even people who really are 80-plus can improve their capacity to perform everyday tasks by becoming more fit.

After you've been doing Quick Fit for a few months, I suggest you take this test again. You'll be surprised and pleased to see how much difference just a daily quarter of an hour can make.

THE KEY ELEMENTS OF QUICK FIT

Quick Fit provides a complete workout with all the essentials of fitness: aerobic activity, strengthening moves, and stretching. You get a bonanza of benefits in just fifteen minutes!

Aerobic Activity

Aerobic means "utilizing oxygen." Aerobic exercise refers to any activity—such as walking, running, swimming, playing basketball—that works the large muscles in your arms and legs, causing you to use more oxygen. During aerobic exercise, your breath quickens and your heart beats more rapidly. Think of it as strength training for your heart, blood vessels, and lungs.

Quick Fit includes ten minutes of aerobic activity. That's enough to make a difference. Aerobic activity is an immediate energizer and mood booster. You'll discover cumulative effects, too. After a few weeks, you'll notice that you have more pep and improved stamina throughout the day. And it's not just a matter of how you feel now: Aerobic exercise is an investment in your future health.

A year and a half ago, I moved from an apartment that had one floor to a house that has two floors. At first, I told my friends, "It's a lot of work living in a house with two floors!" I

used to think about it if I had to go upstairs.
But now, it's no big deal, because I'm in better
shape.

—JANINE

Strengthening Moves

As we head toward age forty, our bodies begin an insidious change. Unless we take preventive measures, we begin to lose muscle and collect additional fat. Even if we don't gain weight, our bodies become less lean. We also lose strength.

Age-related weakness can show up a lot earlier than you might expect. A national survey of more than 16,000 women between ages forty and fifty-five—part of the Study of Women's Health Across the Nation—found that nearly 20 percent of them had difficulty with everyday tasks such as bathing, dressing, carrying groceries, walking, or climbing stairs. An even larger number, 55 percent, reported soreness or stiffness in their necks, backs, or shoulders. Overweight women were twice as likely as those of average weight to report substantial limitations, and they were also more likely to describe aches and pains.

Quick Fit includes four minutes of strengthening exercise. That may not sound like much, but over time, it makes a real difference. Kirsten says:

On Saturdays, from March to December, I work for a
garden plant vendor at an outdoor market. I have to

unload the truck, carry plants around, stand all day sell-
ing them, then load the truck again. In previous years,
when we started up in March, I'd be exhausted after the
first day and my body would ache. But I was amazed to
see that it didn't affect me this year. I'm doing Quick Fit,
so my body is stronger now, and I'm not carrying
around as much weight.

Stretching

Muscles know how to do one thing: Contract. When we lift a
cup to drink, our biceps (a muscle in the front of our upper
arm) contracts. When we lower the cup, another muscle, the
triceps (in the back of our upper arm) contracts to pull our
arm down.

All day long, day after day, our muscles are contracting. If
we don't stretch them out again, over the years we lose flexibility and range of motion. Chronically contracted muscles
cause many of the aches and pains we feel as we get older.
But regular stretching keeps us loose and supple, and helps
prevent the stiffness and discomfort that we might assume
comes from age.

Animals know this instinctively. When a cat wakes up
from a nap, the first thing he does is stretch. He reaches out
his front legs and opens his paws. He arches his back and
extends one back leg and then the other. If it's a really good
stretch, his tail quivers. How ironic that we humans, who
supposedly are creatures of higher intelligence, need to be

told to stretch! Quick Fit includes two flexibility exercises that stretch your muscles from head to toe in just one minute a day.

I'm less stiff in the morning. I have upper back problems, and my back used to feel tired when I woke up. But I haven't noticed that recently.

—PAULINE

IT'S NEVER TOO LATE

Remember those five men who joined the Dallas Bed Rest Study as college students in 1966 and were retested thirty years later? In 1996, their initial checkups showed the physical changes you'd expect to find in middle-aged men. All five of them had gained weight. Four of the men had lost cardiovascular fitness; the one exception was the sole participant who had remained physically active over the past thirty years.

After their preliminary examinations, the five men began rigorous exercise programs. Just six months later, all of them had returned to their 1966 baseline fitness levels. Though in their fifties, they had become just as fit as they were as twenty-year-old college students looking for a summer job. Exercise had turned back the clock.

It's *never* too late to become active and gain remarkable benefit from exercise. Quick Fit can make it happen.

chapter three

WHAT'S HOLDING YOU BACK?

One of our cardinal statistics is that 62 per-cent of the U.S. population acknowledges the benefits of exercise, knows it should exercise more, but never does.
—HARVEY LAUER, PRESIDENT, AMERICAN
SPORTS DATA, INC.

There's a fitness gap in America—and I aim to close it with Quick Fit. On one side, we have the physically active. They're on the streets at 7:00 A.M., jogging and power-walking. They join health clubs and attend exercise classes religiously. They buy treadmills and weight benches, and they actually use them. But a much larger group sits on the other side of the great divide: The Great Sedentary Majority.

Public health officials worry about people who get too little exercise. Their loved ones worry about them—and they worry about themselves. So why don't they get moving? In this chapter, I'll tell you what scientists have found from surveys, as well as what I've learned from years of talking to people about their problems starting and sticking with exercise.

SURVEYING THE SEDENTARY

Every few years a prestigious national organization convenes a committee of leading experts to make exercise recommendations for Americans. These well-qualified professionals review scholarly articles, conduct surveys, and debate new findings. They come up with a brand-new set of exercise guidelines. And then they call a press conference. Their recommendations are always excellent—at least in theory. There's just one problem: Most people don't follow them.

What's holding them back? To find out, the President's Council on Physical Fitness and Sports and the Sporting Goods Manufacturers Association surveyed 1,018 inactive Americans. Guess what: People who don't exercise are well aware of its benefits. Most strongly agree with statements like these:

Even light exercise can improve health and performance.
Exercise reduces tension and stress.
Exercise improves overall quality of life.

Yet they remain inactive. Why? A Council spokesperson summarized the answers in six words: "Too busy, too tired, too lazy."

I have trouble when an exercise program seems to take more time and energy than I have, when it needs equipment, or when I have to go someplace.

—*TINA*

One very encouraging finding from the President's Council's survey is that 59 percent of inactive people would like to change. Among those who were not only sedentary but also concerned about their weight, the number was even higher—74 percent.

The survey findings are consistent with what I hear at the Department of Transportation. I often walk up to people in the hallways and ask, "What are you doing to stay fit?" If they say "Nothing," I ask why.

Occasionally, someone is recovering from an illness or injury, or going through a personal crisis that has put fitness on hold. Sometimes the answers reveal misunderstandings based on lack of good information. For example, one guy told me, "I don't want to use up my allotted heartbeats too soon." No, he wasn't kidding. He simply didn't realize that the heart, like any other muscle, gets stronger with proper use.

Mostly, though, the people I approach say, "I know I need to exercise, but—" and then they explain what's holding them back. We explore the problems and possible solutions. Pretty soon, they realize that it's not impossible after all.

If you truly desire to get fit, you owe it to yourself to list everything that's standing in the way, then to figure out how to move those obstacles aside. Here are the reasons I hear most often—and my suggestions.

> **Not exercising for seven days makes one weak.**

"I DON'T HAVE TIME"

I know you're pressed for time. We all are. We have places to go, people to see, things to do—important things! In the survey of inactive people that I mentioned earlier, the investigators heard over and over: "I would like to exercise more, but I just can't find the time." Seventy-five percent of inactive baby boomers agreed with that statement, as did 76 percent of working women.

All of us have been through personal emergencies that interfere with exercise. If we're committed to staying fit, we return to physical activity when the emergency is over. But some people get derailed. One woman told me that when her daughter gave birth to triplets, she dropped everything to help out. Then she added with a laugh, "The triplets start high school in the fall."

> *Don't look at exercise as just another demand on your time.*
> *Welcome it as a way to get stronger, so you can deal with all the other demands.*

Far more common than these temporary crises is a chronic lack of time. If you're swamped by obligations—job, kids, aging parents, pets, housework, community activities—exercise may be one more thing you simply don't get to. You might even feel guilty about taking time for yourself, whether to read a book or to work out, when you have so many other things to do for everyone else.

If you've been telling yourself for months that you don't have time for exercise, maybe you need to think differently about fitting fitness into your life. If you set aside fifteen minutes of the day to do Quick Fit, you'll still have twenty-three hours and forty-five minutes for everything else you need to get done.

One way to find an extra fifteen minutes is to look for time-stealers. By that I mean any low-priority activity that robs time from a higher priority task, such as exercise. Do any of these time-stealers attack your day?

- Television programs that you don't really enjoy
- Newspaper articles that aren't interesting or useful

- Tedious chitchat at the office water cooler or in online discussion groups
- Video games or Internet surfing that you know is excessive
- Telephone conversations that are longer or more frequent than necessary
- E-mail that takes more time than it's worth

Notice that every single item on this list is something you don't really enjoy or that you consider unimportant. If you could manage to avoid just a few of them, you'd have plenty of time for Quick Fit.

I always have more to do in a day than I can get done. Exercising is easy to "reschedule" for tomorrow. With Quick Fit, it's much harder to do that—I can only fool myself so much. I mean, hey, a ten-minute chunk and a five-minute chunk. Come on, those can fit in somewhere!

—CHUCK

"EXERCISE IS BORING"

Okay, I admit it: Exercise can be boring. If you commute to work, you know that can be boring, too. But it doesn't have to be. I'm sure you know many people—you may be one of them—who turn commuting into a positive part of their day.

They use this time to read or to listen to music, to socialize with friends, or simply to think and daydream. With a little ingenuity, you can do the same with physical activity—I'll elaborate on this suggestion in Chapter 7 (see page 147).

My strategy is to do the walking in the morning while I plan my day and to do the strengthening exercises in the evening while I watch the news. How's that for multitasking?
—PAULINE

"I WAS TRAUMATIZED IN GYM CLASS"

I meet adults who are still hurting from humiliating experiences or cruel comments from decades ago. My best friend in high school and junior high loved sports, but he wasn't athletic. Both of us dreaded the times when the class divided into teams, because we knew he'd be picked last. I'd feel almost as bad as he did. I could see how much it damaged his self-confidence. To me, it seems like a crime to treat a young person in a way that leaves such negative feelings about physical activity.

I hated gym class. You had to be picked for teams, and if you weren't very good at sports, you'd sit there until the very last, feeling

53

rejected. I didn't even want to play—but I wanted to be chosen.

The worst was dodgeball. You were supposed to throw a ball at members of the other team, and they threw it at you. The point was to dodge the ball. It was horrifying for me. I wasn't the kind of kid who wanted to hit and hurt other people. I remember cowering in the corner and being hit by balls that children were throwing with vicious energy.

—TINA

If you're held back by unpleasant school-day memories, give Quick Fit a try. *Anyone* can be good at Quick Fit! This is an equal opportunity exercise program. Grace and talent are not required; you can do this workout with two left feet. Fitness exercise is not gym class. You won't be tested or judged, and there's no competition. You don't even have to worry about achieving your personal best. If you simply show up for your daily workout and get moving, then you're automatically a success.

PHYSICAL EDUCATION FOR ALL!

I'm going to step on my soapbox and tell you what bothers me about most physical education programs: Their emphasis is on sports and competition rather than on lifetime fitness activities like swimming, biking, skating, dancing, and hiking. Little kids love to run around and play games. But high schools and even middle schools and junior highs focus on sports teams. Children must try out for teams, and only a select few get to participate. Everyone else sits in the stadium and watches the game. Because they're spectators, these youngsters begin to assume that physical activity is not for them.

I wish all schools had physical education programs like the Gymkana Troupe, the exhibitional gymnastics team I belonged to when I was at the University of Maryland. Anyone could join. Troupe members came in all sizes and shapes: Tall, short, muscular, pudgy. One of our stars was a very heavy young woman whose specialty was the trampoline. At performances, audiences were startled when she came out in her leotard, because she didn't look like their idea of a gymnast. Sometimes people laughed. But when she finished her routine, with its complex flips and twists, the place would erupt with applause. All of us were so proud of her. We worked hard, encouraged one another, and had a great time. That's what physical education should be.

"I DON'T HAVE THE ENERGY"

When we're wiped out, our first impulse might be to reach for coffee and a snack or to take a nap. But physical activity is actually a terrific pick-me-up. When we move, our heart rate increases and our muscles contract. More blood flows to the brain. Our metabolism is revved up a notch. In short, exercise gets the motor running, and as a result we feel energized.

There's an important bonus for anyone who wants to lose weight: When the workout is finished, the motor keeps running for hours. So the body burns extra calories not only during exercise but even afterward.

I started Quick Fit yesterday. I did my ten-minute walk in the morning. At around nine in the evening I pushed—really pushed—myself to do the remaining five minutes. I told myself that I was too tired. I had a whole bunch of other things to do and I was too tired for any of them. But I did the exercises because I had promised myself I'd start today.

P.S. After I was done, I had the energy to finish all the chores that moments before I was too tired to do.

—ANNE

Try it! The next time you experience that midafternoon or early-evening slump, do Quick Fit. You'll be amazed at how energized you feel.

"I'M TOO OLD"

When someone says to me that they're too old to exercise, I say, "You're too old *not* to exercise." In fact, studies show that seniors well into their eighties and nineties benefit from regular physical activity.

My own father, who will be ninety on his next birthday, is an excellent example. Last spring he developed pneumonia and became so sick that we feared he would die. He was in the hospital for three weeks, then he moved to a nursing home.

When he first arrived at the nursing home, he was too weak to walk. After a few weeks they gave him a walker, but he didn't make much progress with it. I knew his heart was strong, so one day I told him, "Dad, we're going for a walk." I helped him out of his wheelchair, took his hand to help him keep his balance, and we started walking.

On that first day, we walked twenty-five steps, turned around, and walked back to his wheelchair. This took nearly five minutes because we were moving so slowly. The next day we did the same thing, but we walked a few feet farther. After a week, he could walk a hundred steps to the end of the hallway and back again. We kept walking every day, and he progressed. Now my father is doing a lower-intensity version of Quick Fit. We walk for ten minutes, then we go to the rehab room of the nursing home to do the strengthening moves and to stretch. Thanks to daily exercise, my father's quality of life changed dramatically. Instead of being confined to his room, he became mobile.

My mother, who's eighty-one, marveled that my dad was becoming stronger and stronger. I told her, "Of course he is. He's working out every day." A few weeks later, she said, "I want you to put me on that program." So now my mom is doing Quick Fit, too!

Don't let age hold you back. I hope you'll be encouraged to hear that a ninety-year-old guy in a nursing home and his eighty-one-year-old wife can do Quick Fit.

"I'M TOO HEAVY"

In the late 1970s, when I was employed at the YMCA, I worked with a man who weighed 416 pounds. He was thirty-six and lived with his parents; he didn't have a job. He was so large that he couldn't weigh himself on the scale at the Y. If he wanted to check his weight, he went to the nearby Safeway grocery store and the butcher let him use the big meat scale.

We began working together in the spring. Three or four times a week, he arrived at the Y in a van. I knew his legs were strong, because when you weigh 416 pounds, everything you do is weight training. But he couldn't walk two steps without stopping to catch his breath. We didn't talk about his diet (though I encouraged him to see a nutritionist). I just wanted to get him moving. This was years before Quick Fit, so we simply walked. Over the next few months, he managed to work his way up to walking one mile a day. If you don't find that impressive, think what it would be like to walk a mile while carrying a few hundred extra pounds.

By the fall, he had lost one hundred pounds and his life was transformed. He got a job in another state and left the Washington, D.C., area. I think of him every time someone says, "I'm too heavy to exercise."

People who are overweight sometimes get caught in a catch-22 situation concerning fitness. Because they're heavy, exercise is difficult and maybe even painful. Also, they may feel self-conscious about moving, especially if they exercise in public. But of course, it's difficult to lose weight without burning extra calories through physical activity.

Quick Fit is an excellent solution. You can do your workout in the privacy of your own home. You don't have to wear a leotard. The program is short and low intensity, which makes it more tolerable. Yet you'll see significant improvements in fitness over time. Though Quick Fit isn't a weight-loss program, you might lose weight—especially if your success inspires additional exercise and dietary changes, too.

I've lost about eight pounds in eight weeks. It's a combination of Quick Fit, extra walking, and getting a handle on portion size. I know this is a safe way to lose weight, and I feel good about that.

—Bob

"I HATE TO SWEAT"

People hear the word "exercise" and they picture stained T-shirts, necks draped with towels, faces dripping with sweat. For most, it's not an appealing image. Some women tell me they were brought up to believe that perspiring is "unlady-like."

Quick Fit is a no-sweat workout. No sweat means no shower, no change of clothes. In fact, you can complete the entire Quick Fit workout in the time it would take to wash up and get dressed.

One of the things that kept me from exercising before Quick Fit—and it feels ridiculous to admit this—was the need to wear another set of clothes. I'm one of those men who can't stand to go clothes shopping, because I hate to keep taking off and putting on clothes. A midday workout (which is the best time for me, schedule-wise) means getting dressed three times in one day, and, frankly, sometimes I just don't feel like it.

—BOB

"EXERCISE HURTS"

Remember that slogan from the 1980s, "No pain, no gain"? I say, no way! Thank goodness, most fitness experts have abandoned the idea that exercise doesn't count unless it hurts.

Quick Fit is a low-impact exercise program. People rarely experience any discomfort, even at the start. However, if exercise is painful for you, talk to your doctor or a physical therapist. Pain is nature's way of warning us that something is not right. There may be a reason that can be addressed. Or there may be other exercises or modifications of the exercises that would be more comfortable and just as effective for fitness.

"I HAVE MEDICAL PROBLEMS"

Medical problems sometimes interfere with exercise. For instance, you may need to take a break after an injury, during an acute illness, following surgery, or while you're undergoing debilitating medical treatment such as chemotherapy or radiation therapy for cancer.

In the past, people with chronic health problems, such as heart disease, were cautioned against exercise. But we now realize that many of these conditions are not barriers to physical activity. Indeed, the right kind of exercise actually helps. Here are a few examples:

- Heart disease: Physical activity can improve heart health and also counter the disability caused by chronic cardiovascular conditions.
- Lung disease: Physical activity can't reverse damage to the lungs, but it can improve symptoms by helping patients use their lungs more efficiently.
- Diabetes: Exercise combats diabetes by making weight control easier. Also, being fit helps protect against com-

plications, such as heart disease and circulatory problems.

- Arthritis: Though arthritis can make movement painful, well-chosen exercises improve flexibility and reduce pain.
- Osteoporosis: Physical activity helps prevent bone loss. If weakened bones break, exercise helps restore function. Yet another benefit of getting stronger and fitter is improved balance, which reduces the risk of falling.

I had polio as an infant, and there are some residuals; I also have rheumatoid arthritis. I'll never be an athlete. So I appreciate a program that has such simple exercises with aerobic benefit. I think: I've got fifteen minutes. Instead of standing here, I ought to be doing some exercise.

—TONI

If you have these or any other chronic health concerns, discuss exercise with your doctor. You'll probably get a green light, possibly with suggestions for modifying your workout to meet your particular needs.

I used to go to dance classes as often as three times a week. And then things got bad health-

wise. I'd always suffered from headaches, but they went from once or twice a month to five migraines a week, with accompanying nausea.

I had to choose between being medicated into a zombie or really suffering. Dancing class went out the window. I couldn't even do yoga, because I was also having severe neck spasms and pain in my wrists and hands. It's a horrible downward spiral, because the less you move, the worse you feel. My muscle tone diminished; I ended up doing absolutely nothing. I became deeply depressed. I felt so far from my former physically active self. My problems seemed insurmountable.

When I heard about Quick Fit, it touched a nerve. Every other activity seemed depressingly out of reach, which compounded my sense of being powerless over my body. But this seemed like something I could actually succeed at.

—ROWSHANA

"I DON'T WANT TO GO TO A GYM"

You don't have to! You can do Quick Fit at home, at work, or on the road. The whole world is your gym.

I'm a lawyer for an organization within the Department of Transportation. There's lots of congressional interest in what we do, so it can get very busy during the day. I can't set a schedule for going to the gym because if someone from Congress wants something, we have to do it immediately. So I wouldn't necessarily get to a gym at lunchtime or at the end of the day. But I can always fit in fifteen minutes for Quick Fit.

—*CLARE*

"I'M HEALTHY, SO I DON'T NEED TO EXERCISE"

Recently, a slender woman in her early sixties joined the DOT Fitness Center. I asked her what kind of exercise she'd done in the past. "None—I always figured that since I'm not overweight, I didn't have to exercise," she replied. "But now that I'm getting older, I'm losing my strength. I have less energy, and I'm starting to feel creaky, especially in the morning. So I think I need to work out."

How right she is! Fortunately, it's never too late to become physically active.

"I'M LAZY"

No—you're just not motivated to exercise yet. And I aim to change that!

I know all the excuses, because I used them until I ran out. And now I'm here, exercising.
—A DEPARTMENT OF TRANSPORTATION FITNESS
CENTER REGULAR

COMMIT TO GET FIT

When I give seminars on fitness and healthy living, I always spot a few skeptics in the audience. They're leaning back in their chairs, arms folded across their chests, wearing an "I've heard all this before" expression. I run through the benefits of exercise—how it will keep their hearts and lungs strong, help them maintain a healthy weight, make them happier and more productive. The skeptics don't budge. Then I get to Quick Fit. Suddenly, these same people lean forward. Their arms unfold, and they start taking notes.

Toward the end of my seminar, I ask the audience: "If you aren't already exercising consistently, will you start Quick Fit?" Heads nod. Then I ask them to raise their right hands and take a pledge, right there in front of their colleagues or neighbors: "I promise to do the Quick Fit program every day."

Yes, I know this sounds a little corny. Often, there's nervous laughter as the hands go up. But when people give their word, their expressions become more serious. They're determined to begin and to stick with it.

I hope you will commit to Quick Fit. It could be one of the most important commitments of your life. But if you're still at the leaning-back-skeptical stage, that's okay. Would you be willing to do one Quick Fit workout today? Tomorrow, you could make that same choice. I know people who have done Quick Fit for more than three years, without ever making a commitment. One day at a time is what works for them.

You're reading this book because you want to make physical activity part of your daily life. Maybe you've never tried to get fit before. Or perhaps you've been active in the past and somehow went off track. Now you're ready for a fresh start. Quick Fit can make it happen. The program is designed to make exercise so fast and easy that you're bound to succeed.

15 minutes = 900 seconds

THIS TIME WILL BE DIFFERENT

Wouldn't it be great if we could all create healthy new habits on the first try? We'd read an article about good nutrition, and overnight we'd give up candy bars for salad. But as we all know, it takes many attempts to break old habits and create new ones.

Don't be discouraged by the past. All of your previous experiences with exercise—whether positive or negative—have created a foundation upon which you can build future success. Thanks to your earlier efforts, you know more about yourself now than you did before. You've learned what works for you, and what doesn't. That's valuable information, and it will make a difference.

Also, this time you'll be doing Quick Fit. The workout is so simple, it's easy to get started. Staying on track is easy, too, since you can do this program just about anywhere and it takes only fifteen minutes.

FIVE SECRETS OF SUCCESS

Quick Fit is designed for success. Consistency is essential for effective exercise—and consistency requires convenience. By choosing this program, you've already made a significant head start toward a habit of fitness. Here are other ways to stack the odds in your favor.

Secret of Success #1:
Focus on All the Reasons You Want to Exercise

Why do you want to get in shape? Think about everything that makes fitness important to you. The stronger your reasons, the better your chances for success. Motivated people exercise consistently, because they choose to make fitness a priority in their lives.

Many people start exercising to firm up and lose weight. Often, they're inspired by an upcoming landmark birthday, a wedding, a high school reunion, or that annual fitness incentive: Bathing suit season.

Sometimes the reason is an alarming wake-up call, like a heart attack. It doesn't even have to be your own heart attack. One regular at the Department of Transportation Fitness Center joined after his father died of a heart attack at age fifty-seven. Other members in their twenties, thirties, and forties tell me that they're motivated by their parents' poor health. One young man said, "My parents have high blood pressure and diabetes. I see what they're going through because of their lifestyle choices and I want my life to be different."

We asked the people who volunteered to test Quick Fit for this book why they wanted to become more active. Here are some of their answers:

I have a dog and a cat, and I work really hard to keep them healthy. Part of that is making sure they get enough exercise. I realized that I need to take as good care of myself as I do of my pets.

—JANINE

I am healthy and would like to stay that way up to the finish line, if possible. The thing I fear most about old age (I'm sixty-seven) is debility of any kind. I'm working to avoid that. I want to maintain the fullest capacity possible, both mentally and physically, to enjoy life.

— CHUCK

I've been battling depression since my mother's illness and death last year. I had turned into a slug. I used to walk to the library regularly, but I no longer had the energy. Getting out into the fresh air gave me a different outlook for the rest of the day, and I missed that. But part of the depression was feeling that everything was overwhelming. I thought a fifteen-minute program would be a good way to get back into exercise.

— PAULINE

My husband and I hiked in the mountains for our honeymoon last summer. He's very active and fit, and I was getting tired before he did. I just couldn't keep up. There was a particularly *beautiful hike over glaciers, which both of us had been looking forward to. But I realized I couldn't do it. My husband went off and did the hike by himself while I stayed behind. I was so disappointed, especially after we got home and I saw the photographs he took. I was starting to feel like a blob.*

—CLARE

Nine years ago I lost one hundred and eight pounds. I kept it all off for seven years, then my body went into midlife metabolism rebellion. Over the last three years, I've put on about forty of the pounds that I'd kept off so successfully before. Although I'm not trying to get back to my original goal weight now, I do want to stay as healthy as possible. And I don't want my waist size to keep pace with my age!

—BOB

One man I know collected photographs of himself from days when he was in better shape. There's one on his refrigerator, one on his desk at home, and another in his office—reminders of what he'll look like if he sticks with his workouts.

Make a list of all your reasons for exercising and post it

where you'll see it every day. Your own motives to get fit are a potent force. They'll get you started, and they'll keep you going.

Secret of Success #2:
Set Realistic Goals

The other day, a guy told me how frustrated he is because he can't find time for the kind of exercise he wants to do. He said:

> *If I can't work out for at least forty-five minutes, I tell myself, "I'll call it a miss." This happens every day, so I never do even a little bit of exercise.*

I sympathized with his frustration but urged him not to be so hard on himself. Forty-five minutes is an impressive goal. However, *any* amount of exercise is better than none.

Some folks assume that exercise has to be "challenging." So they make fitness difficult for themselves. Some health clubs offer workouts based on marine boot camp. Now *that's* challenging! But what happens when people begin a very demanding program, one that requires a lot of time or painful effort? Most of them just can't stick with it. Even the real marine boot camp at Parris Island lasts just twelve weeks, and I've never met a marine who wished it had continued longer.

Quick Fit is different. This program makes exercise as

easy as possible. It's designed for lifelong fitness, not temporary boot camp. The priority here is consistency. When exercise is easy, so is success.

Secret of Success #3:
Schedule Exercise into Your Day

Is your workout on your To Do List? We schedule all the things we consider important, plus so much more. But too often, exercise is left out. We think, "I'll squeeze it in." Or, if we remember to put it on the list, it comes after everything else, at the end of the day. And often we simply can't get to it.

> **You can start to exercise now**
> **to avoid a heart attack.**
> **Or you can wait to exercise**
> **until after you have a heart attack—**
> **if you survive it.**

Fitness doesn't seem like an emergency. If it did, we'd drop everything else and work out. But lack of fitness could lead to an emergency. If exercise is truly important to you, it's worth scheduling into your day. Even the president of the United States finds time for a daily workout—and we'd all agree that the president is a busy person.

If you're committed to following the Quick Fit program,

start by figuring out exactly when you will do your workouts. The more easily you can slip exercise into your day, the more likely that you'll do it consistently. Some suggestions:

Harness the Power of Habit

Some people reinvent their exercise program every day. They ask questions like: "What should I do?" and "When should I start?" Then they negotiate with themselves: "Do I have to do it now? I'm not in the mood. Besides, I really need to return that phone call."

So what happens? Exercise is postponed. The phone call is made. Then something else comes up. After a whole day of "I'll do it later," bedtime arrives and the workout never happened. But think how much mental time and energy have been wasted—and how discouraging it is to have nothing to show for it.

Exercise is so much easier if it's a habit. You don't have to make any decisions; there's nothing to negotiate. You don't have to talk yourself into it. You just do it automatically, day after day. Over time, working out becomes comfortable and familiar. You may actually miss exercise if something interferes with your routine.

The easiest way to establish an exercise habit is to link your Quick Fit workout to something else you already do every day. Some people come to the Department of Transportation Fitness Center during their coffee break as faithfully as they used to stop by the snack machines. Others do Quick Fit every day for the first fifteen minutes of their lunch hour.

Here are examples from the people who tested the program for this book. As you'll see, they had very different preferences. But they succeeded with Quick Fit at all hours of the day:

I have found that I exercise best at night. So, I have been doing Quick Fit while I watch the news, or Wheel of Fortune, *or* Jeopardy.

—ANNE

I don't have the energy or desire to exercise first thing in the morning. When I first get up, I want to have my coffee, get myself in front of the computer, and start doing some work. I also don't want to exercise on a full stomach, so right after lunch is out. And by the middle-to-late afternoon, I'm more ready for a nap than a walk on the treadmill! So, before lunch just seems to be the best time.

—BOB

I'm addicted. No matter what's going on at work, every morning at nine I go to the Fitness Center. Coworkers know they can't make nine o'clock appointments with me. I

*spend fifteen minutes in the gym, then I get a
skim latte and go back to my desk.*

— K*IRSTEN*

---

*My work style is that once I get going, I really
don't like to stop. I found it helped me to work
out first thing in the morning. This way, exercise doesn't interfere. By the time I wake up
and figure out I don't want to work out, I'm
already done.*

— N*ANCY*

Look at your own schedule—or your schedules, if week-
ends and weekdays are different—and figure out what's best
for you. Even if your days are mostly unpredictable, you can
probably find a spot on which to build a routine.

Write down everything that you do daily without fail. The
list may be short:

1. Wake up
2. Go to sleep.

But perhaps you can add to it. Do you predictably—

- Fetch the newspaper from outside the front door?
- Check e-mail?
- Commute to work?

- Listen to a favorite radio or TV program?
- Drive kids to school or to appointments?
- Eat breakfast, lunch, or dinner?
- Take a coffee break?
- Telephone an elderly parent?
- Shower?
- Nap?

Now look at your list. Is there any daily activity you could combine with Quick Fit? That's a great way to fit in exercise: You don't have to disrupt your normal routine, and you don't need to spend any extra time. For example:

- Do you watch the news or another TV show every day? If so, instead of sitting in your favorite chair through the whole program, why not do Quick Fit for the first fifteen minutes? You won't even notice that you're exercising.
- Could you work the ten-minute walk into your commute? One possibility is to get off the bus or train one stop early and walk the rest of the way. Another is to park in a more remote location.
- Do you play with your kids? If your children, like many of today's youngsters, aren't getting enough physical activity, a brisk family walk would be quality time in more ways than one.

If combining exercise with something else doesn't work, what about tucking Quick Fit into the time just before a regular activity? Perhaps you could do Quick Fit while your computer is booting up and collecting your e-mail. If you pick up kids at school, could you arrive ten minutes early and take a walk on the track?

As you think about your schedule, ask yourself if Quick Fit could help you through a predictably difficult time of the day. Many people use exercise to counter their usual midafternoon slump. Or they clear their minds and reduce stress by working out after work.

I hope you will find a time that works well for you. That's a key part of making exercise easy to do.

Consider the Case for Morning Exercise

The best time for your Quick Fit workout is whatever time you'll do it consistently. That's the bottom line. However, studies suggest that most people are more consistent when they exercise in the morning. This doesn't surprise me. I exercise at 6:30 A.M. every day, even when I'm on vacation. My workout jump-starts me for the day. The fresh air clears my mind; I make plans. Later, various demands will compete for my time. But during these special minutes, nothing interrupts me.

> *If you exercise first thing in the morning, it doesn't matter what else comes up during the day—meetings, phone calls, emergencies. Nothing can interfere with a workout that's already finished.*

I realize that morning exercise isn't for everyone. You may be a working parent whose mornings are already overloaded getting the kids ready for school or child care. Or you might be one of those night owls for whom it's a challenge just to boil water for coffee in the morning. But if you've had difficulty sticking with exercise in the past, and have never started your day with a workout, give it a try just once. Even if you're not a "morning person," physical activity will get your blood circulating and give you an energy boost. You'll feel great going through the entire day knowing that you've already done your exercise.

The reason I don't exercise isn't because I don't want to; I do. I don't exercise because I schedule it at the end of the day, and I never get to it.

—A DOT FITNESS CENTER REGULAR, WHO NOW COMES AT 7:00 A.M.

Expect the Unexpected

Even the best routines can break down. So you need a Plan B. If your walk is rained out, what will you do instead? How will you arrange for your daily Quick Fit workout if your in-laws arrive for a week or if you take a holiday in Las Vegas? A little advance planning usually allows you to stay consistent with exercise. In Chapter 7, I'll give you some suggestions for doing Quick Fit when you're away from home, including tips on keeping up with strength training, without having to lug heavy dumbbells.

When exercise is disrupted temporarily, try to get back to your workout routine as quickly as possible. You will probably find—as I have—that physical activity is a real lifeline when everything else in your life seems out of control.

Secret of Success #4: Line Up Support

If you were a professional athlete, you'd have an entourage: Coaches, assistants, workout partners, fans. As a person who is about to develop a consistent exercise habit, you deserve no less. Don't try to go it alone.

Tell the World You're Starting Quick Fit

When you begin an exercise program, do you keep it to yourself? Many people do. They figure that if they don't say anything, no one will know if they quit. That's why I suggest you do exactly the opposite. And when I say "tell the world," I really mean it!

Tell your family and your friends. But don't stop there. Tell your boss and your colleagues at work; mention it to your neighbors. Let your doctor and other health care providers know. The more people you tell, the more motivated you will be to stay consistent. Plus, talking about Quick Fit helps you gain additional support.

QUICK FIT

Ask for Encouragement

We all need cheerleaders in our lives. Becoming consistent about exercise is a challenge. Ask your family and friends to applaud your efforts. People who care about you will be happy that you're doing something good for your health.

Request Practical Help, If You Need It

Quick Fit is so simple that you might not require any assistance. But perhaps you could use a helping hand to set up your workout space. Or maybe you have little kids who suddenly require attention the minute you pick up a dumbbell. Don't hesitate to ask for what you need in order to work out.

Form a Team

Quick Fit is contagious: If you talk about it, and if others see you doing it, the next thing you know, family members, neighbors, and colleagues will want to join you. And that's great news, because exercise is a lot more fun with friends.

Some of the most successful members of the Department of Transportation Fitness Center are the ones who have formed fitness teams. I'm talking about the people who are most consistent, not the best athletes. Teams don't compete; members work out together and cheer one another on. When colleagues are doing Quick Fit together, no one wants to let the others down.

With some of the DOT teams, you couldn't skip a workout even if you wanted to. One guy told his team that he was too tired to exercise that day. He left his office for a minute, and while he was gone, a couple of his buddies hid his chair. When he got back, they delivered an ultimatum: "If you don't work out, you can't sit down." He laughed and joined them at the Fitness Center.

Secret of Success #5: Make Your Workouts Fun

Have a good time while you get in shape. Your body will benefit just as much if you do Quick Fit while watching TV, listening to lively music, or chatting with a friend.

Another approach is to treat exercise as a respite during the day. People often tell me, "My workout is time for me." They see it as a minivacation.

I exercise to get away from the telephone, the cell phone, the fax, and the copier machine.
—OVERHEARD AT THE
DOT FITNESS CENTER

START TODAY

When I buy something new and different—whether it's a pair of shoes or a golf club—I can't wait to try it out. I hope you feel just as excited about Quick Fit, because the best time to start exercising is right now.

You don't have to wait until Monday. You don't have to start on your birthday, on the first day of the month, or on New Year's Day. You don't even have to wait until you've read this entire book. Quick Fit is so simple that you can start immediately. See pages 101–102 for a plan that lets you jump right to the instructions. (And see pages 214–215 if you're not quite ready to begin.)

Now, let's get moving!

GETTING READY FOR SUCCESS

You've made a commitment to begin Quick Fit. A few things remain to be done before you start. This chapter walks you through the preliminaries.

You'll take a simple test to see if you need medical clearance for exercise. Next, you'll need to figure out when and where to do Quick Fit. A big part of getting ready for success is doing everything possible to make exercise convenient. I'll suggest how to set up a workout spot and assemble the gear you need. Then you'll be ready to begin.

If you're impatient to get going, skip to the end of this chapter (pages 101–102) and read Quick Start, a guide to starting Quick Fit immediately.

DO YOU NEED MEDICAL CLEARANCE?

I'm sure you've read the advice about getting your doctor's permission before you begin a vigorous exercise program. I've always thought people should be required to obtain medical clearance if they want to be sedentary and out of shape. "Doc," they'd say, "I'm planning to skip exercise and grow my gut. Whaddya think?" Can you imagine the response?

Quick Fit is moderate, not vigorous, exercise. Nevertheless, you need to check with your health care provider if:

- You are age seventy or older
- You are pregnant or might be pregnant
- You have any medical condition that could make it necessary to modify the Quick Fit program

To find out if this precaution applies to you, take the PAR-Q (see box, page 87). This test, devised by the Canadian Society for Exercise Physiology, is widely used to screen people who are planning to begin an exercise program.

Even if you have no cause for concern, I encourage you to establish a relationship with your doctor. Make an appointment if your routine checkup is overdue. Some people skip their annual physical. They're too busy. Or they're afraid they won't like what they hear. But a medical exam can be an excellent source of motivation. Later, the results will help you measure your progress. Think how encouraged you'll be when you see what a year of Quick Fit does for those blood pressure and cholesterol numbers.

Physical Activity Readiness
Questionnaire - PAR-Q
(revised 2002)

PAR-Q & YOU

(A Questionnaire for People Aged 15 to 69)

Regular physical activity is fun and healthy, and increasingly more people are starting to become more active every day. Being more active is very safe for most people. However, some people should check with their doctor before they start becoming much more physically active.

If you are planning to become much more physically active than you are now, start by answering the seven questions in the box below. If you are between the ages of 15 and 69, the PAR-Q will tell you if you should check with your doctor before you start. If you are over 69 years of age, and you are not used to being very active, check with your doctor.

Common sense is your best guide when you answer these questions. Please read the questions carefully and answer each one honestly: check YES or NO.

YES	NO		
☐	☐	1.	Has your doctor ever said that you have a heart condition <u>and</u> that you should only do physical activity recommended by a doctor?
☐	☐	2.	Do you feel pain in your chest when you do physical activity?
☐	☐	3.	In the past month, have you had chest pain when you were not doing physical activity?
☐	☐	4.	Do you lose your balance because of dizziness or do you ever lose consciousness?
☐	☐	5.	Do you have a bone or joint problem (for example, back, knee or hip) that could be made worse by a change in your physical activity?
☐	☐	6.	Is your doctor currently prescribing drugs (for example, water pills) for your blood pressure or heart condition?
☐	☐	7.	Do you know of <u>any other reason</u> why you should not do physical activity?

If

you

answered

YES to one or more questions

Talk with your doctor by phone or in person BEFORE you start becoming much more physically active or BEFORE you have a fitness appraisal. Tell your doctor about the PAR-Q and which questions you answered YES.

- You may be able to do any activity you want — as long as you start slowly and build up gradually. Or, you may need to restrict your activities to those which are safe for you. Talk with your doctor about the kinds of activities you wish to participate in and follow his/her advice.
- Find out which community programs are safe and helpful for you.

NO to all questions

If you answered NO honestly to <u>all</u> PAR-Q questions, you can be reasonably sure that you can:
- start becoming much more physically active – begin slowly and build up gradually. This is the safest and easiest way to go.
- take part in a fitness appraisal – this is an excellent way to determine your basic fitness so that you can plan the best way for you to live actively. It is also highly recommended that you have your blood pressure evaluated. If your reading is over 144/94, talk with your doctor before you start becoming much more physically active.

→

DELAY BECOMING MUCH MORE ACTIVE:
- if you are not feeling well because of a temporary illness such as a cold or a fever – wait until you feel better; or
- if you are or may be pregnant – talk to your doctor before you start becoming more active.

PLEASE NOTE: If your health changes so that you then answer YES to any of the above questions, tell your fitness or health professional. Ask whether you should change your physical activity plan.

<u>Informed Use of the PAR-Q</u>: The Canadian Society for Exercise Physiology, Health Canada, and their agents assume no liability for persons who undertake physical activity, and if in doubt after completing this questionnaire, consult your doctor prior to physical activity.

Source: Physical Activity Readiness Questionnaire (PAR-Q), copyright 2002. Reprinted with permission from the Canadian Society for Exercise Physiology. *http://www.csep.ca/forms.asp*

WHEN AND WHERE?

Scheduling your workout is the key to making it happen. Ideally, you'll plan to do Quick Fit at a time that fits easily into your daily routine. Chapter 4 offered many suggestions (see pages 74–81).

Once you know *when,* figure out *where* you'll do your workouts. Quick Fit is so flexible that it can be done nearly anywhere. If there's a fitness room where you work or live, bingo. But if you're thinking about joining a health club over in the next town and doing the exercises there, forget it! Quick Fit is designed to make fitness easy so that nothing stops you from being consistent. An inconvenient workout spot is not in the spirit of Quick Fit.

A Place for Aerobic Exercise

Quick Fit calls for ten minutes of aerobic activity. Either you'll take a ten-minute walk—which can be done on a treadmill or outdoors—or you'll do an indoor aerobic exercise routine. The Quick Fit indoor routine can be done in the same small space you'll use for the strengthening and stretching exercises.

If You're Using a Treadmill

Do you have convenient access to a motorized treadmill? If so, begin Quick Fit with that. Treadmills have cushioned decks that put a spring in your step while protecting your joints from the pounding they'd get on cement. The walking surface is dry and even, so you're less likely to slip or trip. And your daily walk will never get rained out. A motorized treadmill keeps a steady pace. Most can be set to signal that your ten minutes are up. All this helps you stay consistent. I'll have more to say about treadmills below when I discuss equipment.

If You Plan to Walk Outdoors

Figure out a walking place that's safe—that's the number one consideration. The other key issue is convenience. Let's be realistic: It doesn't make much sense to get into the car and drive fifteen minutes to reach the perfect spot for a ten-minute walk. You'll be doing Quick Fit every day. The ideal outdoor walking place is just out the front door at home or at work, or at some appropriate spot that you pass daily as part of your normal routine. Avoid routes that involve crossing busy streets or dodging crowds, because they'll slow you down.

A Place for Strengthening and Stretching

Set up a workout area. A corner of your bedroom, living room, or office will do. Quick Fit's strengthening exercises and stretches—as well as the indoor aerobic routine—can be done in any clear space about four feet wide by six feet long. Select an area that's easy to keep clutter-free.

Since three of the exercises are performed on the floor, you'll be more comfortable if your workout space is carpeted. Otherwise, pad the floor with a mat or towel. You'll be timing the exercises, so a clock that displays minutes and seconds is useful. If entertainment would make your sessions more enjoyable, find room for a TV, radio, or CD player. Put all your Quick Fit gear—a copy of this book, your weights, a rolled-up mat or towel if you use them, a water bottle if you like—on a nearby shelf or in a handy container.

Some people take pains to make their workout area appealing as well as convenient. They post pictures and inspirational sayings; they position themselves so they can see an attractive view. All this helps sustain motivation.

EQUIPMENT

Once you've decided upon a place for your Quick Fit workouts, assemble your equipment and learn how to use it safely.

Treadmill

You may already own or have access to a treadmill. According to a 2001 survey conducted by American Sports Data, 41.6 million Americans use treadmills to stay fit. They are the most popular type of aerobic exercise equipment by far.

If you aren't yet familiar with treadmills, take a few minutes to learn the basics (see box). Some treadmills look like control panels for jet airplanes. Built into them are elaborate computerized programs that guide you through specialized workouts, such as programs that simulate running up and down hills.

Forget about all that! For Quick Fit, all you need to know is how to make the treadmill move at three miles per hour.

Very important: If you have children or pets, make sure they're safely away from the treadmill when you're using it. Between workouts, keep the treadmill locked or unplugged so that a youngster can't start it without your supervision.

FIRST TIME ON A TREADMILL?

Before you get on the treadmill for the first time, stand next to it and learn how it works. Look for the buttons that make the treadmill go faster or slower. See if it's possible to time your workout. Locate the Stop button, just in case you ever need to end your workout in a hurry. Once you're acquainted with the controls, turn off the treadmill. You're ready to take your first walk:

- After the belt stops moving, get on the treadmill and straddle the belt. Stand on the stationary frame, with one foot on the left side of the belt and one foot on the right side.
- Start the treadmill at its slowest speed. Look down at the belt to make sure that it's moving slowly.
- Hold on to the side or front railing and step onto the belt. Begin walking. The pace will be slow.
- When you're completely accustomed to the experience of walking on a treadmill, increase the speed very slightly. Gradually work your way up to a speed that's comfortable but brisk (three miles per hour is standard for Quick Fit).

- While you walk, keep at least one hand on the railing for balance. Look straight ahead. If you need to turn, first grip the handrail with both hands. Otherwise, you might lose your balance.
- After your walk, hold on to the treadmill as it stops. Take a few seconds to regain your "land legs" before you step onto the floor.

Working with Weights

Three of Quick Fit's strengthening exercises are done with a pair of light dumbbells. The weight to use depends upon your strength. Remember that question in Chapter 2 about whether you can lift a heavy suitcase into an overhead compartment?

- If you answered "Yes," buy a pair of five-pounders.
- If you answered "No," ask yourself another question: What if it was a heavy purse instead of a suitcase—could you lift that into an overhead compartment? If you could manage the purse, buy three-pound dumbbells.
- If you couldn't lift a purse into an overhead compartment, buy one-pound weights—or use one-pound cans, provided you can hold them easily.

Most men start with five-pound weights; most women start with threes. When you become stronger, you may want to move up to heavier weights. I'll explain how to do that in Chapter 7 (see pages 158–159).

Where to Buy Weights

Strength training is so popular these days that dumbbells are sold at most discount stores. Shops that specialize in exercise equipment offer a variety of styles and colors. Check your local Yellow Pages under "Sporting Goods."

Expect to pay $5 to $15 for a pair of dumbbells, depending on the style and weight. That's not much for equipment that lasts a lifetime. Least expensive are the plain gray cast-iron type, with hexagonal ends. That's the kind I have. They usually cost about 50 cents a pound, which is cheaper than chicken. But you might prefer to splurge on colorful plastic-coated versions. Avoid dumbbells with round ends, because even a three-pound weight can do damage if it rolls off a table and lands on your foot. Ouch!

If you'd rather shop online or by telephone, and have the weights delivered to your door, below are a few possibilities. Warning: Shipping will cost about as much as the dumbbells themselves.

- Fitness Wholesale: 895-A Hampshire Road, Stow, OH 44224 888-FW-ORDER or 330-929-7227; *http://www.fit nesswholesale.com*
- MC Sports: 3070 Shaffer Avenue, SE, Grand Rapids, MI 49512 616-942-2600 or 888-801-9159; *http://www.mcsports.com*
- Fitness First: PO Box 251, Shawnee Mission, KS 66201 800-421-1791; *http://www.fitness1st.com*

Weight Safety

Light dumbbells are one of the safest types of exercise equipment. Nevertheless, they must be treated with respect.

- Store your dumbbells in a safe place, so that no one trips on them. If you have young children, keep the weights out of reach. Curious youngsters might hurt themselves (or your floors) if they drop a dumbbell.
- Pick up your weights carefully: Bend at the knees for balance and support, and use your leg power to rise. Even though these are light dumbbells, if you store a couple of pairs in the same tote bag, and then try to lift the bag with one hand, it won't feel light!
- If possible, store your weights at waist height, to prevent back strain when you're picking them up. I use a dumbbell rack, so I don't have to lean over to grab my weights.
- After your workout, move just as carefully as you put your weights away.

COME AS YOU ARE

You won't get sweaty with Quick Fit, so you don't need special exercise clothes for this program. Wear any outfit that doesn't restrict your movement. If you can walk, stretch, and lie down on the floor, you're dressed for success with Quick Fit. At the Department of Transportation Fitness Center, most people do the program in business attire.

Sometimes they remove jackets, ties, scarves, and jewelry, but that's it.

BEST FOOT FORWARD

Quick Fit requires no special shoes. Some women at DOT do the program in heels, though I advise against this. Why risk a sprained ankle or a fall? Better to go for comfort. These days, you don't have to decide between attractive and comfortable. You can easily find shoes that feel as good as they look.

Wearing comfortable shoes is important all the time, not just during the fifteen minutes of your Quick Fit workout. When your feet hurt, everything hurts. Ask yourself these questions:

- Do you frequently develop blisters on your feet?
- Do your feet sometimes need a break when you're walking— say, on a shopping trip or a museum visit?
- Does walking cause pain in your ankles, knees, or back?

If the answer to all three questions is "No," you can assume you're wearing shoes that fit properly. In that case, you can skip the rest of this section. But come back if your feet start bothering you when you become more active with Quick Fit.

Walking shouldn't hurt! Discuss any chronic problems with your doctor or podiatrist. There are many reasons for foot, ankle, knee, or back pain, and some of these require medical treatment. But the culprit could be improper footwear. You'd be amazed at the difference the right shoes can make.

Fit to Be Tied

Too many people walk around like Cinderella's stepsisters, their feet crammed into shoes that don't fit. A survey by the American Orthopaedic Foot and Ankle Society found that nearly 90 percent of women wore shoes that were too small. As a result, about 80 percent of them had foot problems. Interestingly, men are much less likely to select shoes that are too small.

Ladies: Are you still wearing the same size shoe that you wore in high school? Even if you can still fit into the same dress size, your feet probably are longer and wider than they were when you were a teenager.

Do yourself a favor: Go to a real shoe store, the kind with experienced sales people, and have your feet measured. Yes, *feet*—both of them. Many people have feet that are not the same size. Shoes should be fitted to the larger foot; if necessary, an insert can be used to make the smaller foot match the other shoe.

Time your visit to the shoe store for the afternoon or evening, because your feet expand during the day. Wear the kind of socks you'll wear for exercise. If you normally use orthotics (corrective shoe inserts), bring them along. Also bring a well-worn pair of shoes. The pattern of wear will tell the salesperson what you need. For example, if wear is uneven, you may need shoes that stabilize your feet in the proper position. Always try on both shoes—unless you plan to just hop on one foot.

INTERESTING SHOE-FITTING FACT

The T-shaped chrome and black gizmo that shoe stores use to measure your feet is called the Brannock Device. It's named for Charles Brannock, who invented it in 1927. The factory he founded still manufactures them in Syracuse, New York.

The Brannock Device measures the length of your foot from heel to toe; the width of your foot at the ball; and the length of your arch, the ball-to-heel measurement. All three numbers are needed to determine proper fit.

Give new shoes a test-drive before you buy them:

- Stand up. Move your toes. Do they have plenty of wriggle room? Good. Toes shouldn't touch the front of the shoe.
- Walk. Make sure your heel and foot don't slide inside the shoe. If shoes are too big, you're more likely to develop blisters and to lose your balance.
- Walk some more. Take a few minutes to see how the shoes feel. Does anything pinch? If so, find another pair. Shoes should feel comfortable right out of the box. Forget about breaking them in. If shoes don't fit properly, they'll break in your feet.

These Shoes Were Made for Walking

When I was growing up, there were shoes and there were sneakers. All sneakers looked alike, except for the colors. These days you can hardly find plain sneakers. Instead, you see a bewildering array of walking shoes, running shoes, cross-training shoes, and shoes for every sport. There's a point to this variety. Running and other sports are harder on the feet than walking is, so specialty shoes are more cushioned. They also feature stabilizing devices designed to keep the foot well positioned even when it's slamming against the pavement or meeting other sport-specific challenges.

What kind of shoe should you get for Quick Fit? For most people, a comfortable walking shoe is best. To a walker, a running shoe may feel bulky or overly rigid. However, if your feet need pampering, or if they have a tendency to roll when you walk (see box on pronating and supinating), a running shoe might be better. A competent shoe salesperson can help you make the right choice.

ARE YOU A PRONATER OR A SUPINATOR?

This is not a question about politics! I'm asking if your feet tend to roll inward (pronate) or roll outward (supinate) when you walk. Feet normally do both. First, you land on your heel. Your foot is designed to pronate as you move forward. This flattens the arch, allowing the entire bottom of your foot to absorb the impact when you land on the ground. Then, as you push off from your toes to complete the step, your foot supinates.

Many people pronate or supinate too much. This can lead to pain in the feet, ankles, legs, and even in the hips or back. One simple way to tell if you might have a problem is to examine your shoes for uneven wear:

- Look at the wear pattern on the soles. If there's more wear on the inside, that's a sign of pronation; excess wear on the outside of the sole may be caused by supination.

- Check the heels. They normally become worn on the outside. But excessive wear on the inside suggests pronation.

- Put your shoes on a shelf at eye level, with the backs toward you. If they tilt inward, you may pronate too much; if they tilt outward, that could indicate excess supination.

A podiatrist can check your gait and recommend shoes or orthotics that can control pronation or supination, making walking more comfortable.

Keeping Your Feet Happy

If you're sedentary, your exercise footwear languishes in the closet. But once you start Quick Fit, you're putting half a mile a day on your shoes, or three and a half miles a week. That's the equivalent of a marathon every couple of months—more if you become more active, as so many people do after they start this program. For the first time in your life, you may wear out your shoes!

You can't always tell that your shoes are worn out, especially if you exercise indoors. Your shoes could look clean and unscuffed on the outside even if the cushioning on the inside is feeling its age. For that reason, experts advise that you keep track of the miles, just as you do to know when your car needs an oil change.

The standard advice is to replace your walking shoes every 300 to 500 miles. If all you're using those shoes for is Quick Fit—half a mile and then you take them off for the day——you'd need a new pair every two years. But if your feet or legs begin to hurt, it could be time for new shoes, even if you haven't yet reached 300 miles. Look at the heel and sole. My motto: When there's obvious wear, you need a new pair.

Now that you've gotten in gear, you're ready to roll with Quick Fit. Next, you'll learn the moves. One approach is to read Chapter 6, which takes you through the entire program step-by step. But if you'd rather begin immediately, learning as you go, just use Quick Start (see next page).

> *You have the skill—*
> *now add the will.*
> *Start exercising today*
> *and enjoy the rest of your life,*
> *strong and fit!*

QUICK START FOR QUICK FIT

The best time to start exercising is *now*. If you can't finish the entire book today, use the instructions below to begin Quick Fit immediately.

Here's the plan:

- **PAR-Q:** Take the PAR-Q (see page 87), a test to see if you need medical clearance to do Quick Fit. It takes only a minute to complete. Call your doctor if necessary—that's progress, too. Otherwise, begin exercising.

- **AEROBIC ACTIVITY:** Do ten minutes of aerobic activity. Move at a pace that feels brisk but manageable. If you can't sing one line of a song in a single breath while you're exercising (e.g., "Take me out to the ball game" or "I've been working on the railroad"), slow down. Here are three options, no learning required:

    OPTION #1: If you have access to a treadmill and have used it before, take a ten-minute treadmill walk. Go at your own speed, aiming for three miles per hour.

    OPTION #2: If you like to walk outdoors, do that briskly for ten minutes.

    OPTION #3: Put on some music and dance, walk indoors, or march in place for ten minutes. Or try Quick Steps (pages 110–117).

The aerobic activity is two-thirds of the Quick Fit workout. Add the rest now. Or add one exercise per day to learn the program in a week.

To learn the strengthening exercises and stretches: Read the instructions, just a few pages for each exercise. Or ask a friend to read them aloud while you do the moves— it's like having a personal trainer.

ABDOMINAL CRUNCH (pages 122–126): This exercise is performed on the floor. If getting down on the floor is difficult, see the instructions on pages 205–206. Or simply do this and the other floor exercises while lying on a bed (see pages 206–207).

BICEPS CURL (pages 128–130): Most women start with three-pound dumbbells; most men use five-pounders. Too heavy? No dumbbells? Use one-pound cans instead.

FLOOR BENCH PRESS (pages 131–133)

STANDING ROW (pages 134–136)

SIDE BEND (pages 137–139)

SIT AND REACH (pages 140–142)

Congratulations! You've learned Quick Fit and you've begun to exercise. Read the book when you have time. Meanwhile, keep up the good work!

THE QUICK FIT PROGRAM

In this chapter, I'll take you through the Quick Fit work-out step by step. At the end, on pages 144–145, you'll find a double-page summary that shows you the entire program at a glance, in words and pictures. After you've learned the moves, you can use this summary for a quick reminder.

Your workout begins with ten minutes of aerobic activity. A brisk walk will do the trick, but I'll give you another option if you'd rather not go outdoors and don't have access to a treadmill. Your walk gets your heart pumping and warms up your muscles. This prepares you for the strengthening exer-cises.

Next, you'll tackle your midsection with a one-minute abdominal exercise.

After that, you'll complete three exercises that address the muscles in your upper body, spending a total of about three minutes.

You've been contracting your muscles, so your workout ends with two stretches—one for the lower body, one for the upper body—to lengthen them out again. You'll stretch for one minute.

That's it! There's no need to warm up or cool down, since Quick Fit is no-sweat exercise. You'll do this workout every day, because consistency is the name of the game. Remember, it's just a quarter of an hour, no longer than a coffee break.

"MUST I DO THE ENTIRE QUICK FIT WORKOUT AT ONCE?"

Someone always asks this question when I give a talk about Quick Fit, and it always gets a laugh. You'd think that a fifteen-minute program would be short enough. But it may make sense for you to break up the workout. And yes, it's fine to do the ten-minute aerobic portion at one time and the strengthening exercises and stretches (which take five minutes) at another. I don't recommend subdividing the program further than that: Keeping track of your workout would become complicated, and the whole point of Quick Fit is to make fitness simple.

Some people at the Department of Transportation do their strengthening exercises and stretches at home, either first thing in the morning or in the evening while they're watching TV. Then, during their lunch break, they go outside for a ten-minute walk or they come to the Fitness Center and walk on the treadmill.

The best schedule
is the one that makes it easiest
for you to remain consistent.

INDIVIDUALIZING YOUR WORKOUT

Quick Fit was designed to be suitable for individuals of all ages, shapes, and sizes—from slender women in their twenties, to overweight middle-aged men, to senior citizens. Nevertheless, the regular program may be too difficult or too easy for you. Therefore, the instructions include suggestions for customizing the exercises.

If you have chronic or temporary physical limitations—or if you've been very sedentary—and you can't manage regular Quick Fit, start with the Quick Fit Lite version. Over time, you'll become stronger and your endurance will increase. Follow the instructions to work your way up to regular Quick Fit, if possible.

On the other hand, if you're already physically active and plan to use Quick Fit only as a supplement, the regular program may be insufficiently challenging. Use Quick Fit Plus instead. Or you might decide to work up to Quick Fit Plus after doing regular Quick Fit for a while. All three versions take just fifteen minutes; the only difference is the intensity of the exercises.

IMPORTANT CAUTION

Quick Fit is designed to be safe for your heart. But if you experience any of these symptoms, *stop immediately and contact your doctor for advice*:

- Pain, tightness, or pressure in your chest
- Unexplained pain in your arm, shoulder, or jaw
- Difficulty breathing or extreme shortness of breath
- Dizziness or light-headedness
- Profuse sweating
- Nausea

PART 1: AEROBIC ACTIVITY

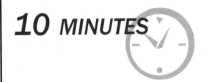

10 MINUTES

You have three options for aerobic activity: Treadmill walking, outdoor walking, or a low-impact aerobic routine, called Quick Steps, which can be done in a corner of your home or office. You'll find additional suggestions in Chapter 7—take your pick, or combine them. For example, you might walk on the treadmill during the week if there's a fitness center where you work. Then over the weekend, you could hit the pavement in your neighborhood, switching to the indoor aerobic routine in bad weather.

Your Heart Rate Never Lies

Your heart is always pumping, but the rate varies considerably, depending on what you're doing. When you snooze in an easy chair, the rate slows; when you get up and move around, your heart beats more quickly. Since your heart automatically keeps pace with your physical effort, your heart rate tells you how hard you're working.

An aerobic workout should make your heart beat faster—but not too fast. How do you know that you're exercising at the right intensity? One way is to figure out your target heart rate, the age-adjusted rate that's appropriate for aerobic activity, then measure your actual heart rate and compare the two. I'll tell you how to do that in Chapter 7 (see pages 155–158). But this simple song test is all you really need:

While you're moving, start singing. Pretend you're in the shower. When you're exercising at the right intensity for Quick Fit, you should be able to sing one line in a single breath. For example:

"Take me out to the ball game" or
"Row, row, row your boat" or
"Hail, hail, the gang's all here."

If you need to take a breath in the middle of the line, slow down! But if you can sing not only the first line but also the second, then you could move faster without taxing your heart and lungs. Unless you have some other physical limitation, pick up the pace a little, especially if you're walking at less than three miles per hour or if your goal is a more challenging workout.

Customizing Your Walking Workout

It's simple to customize a walk: Just adjust the speed!

Quick Fit Lite: If three miles per hour is too fast, start at whatever pace is comfortable for you. Gradually work your way up to three miles per hour. Most people can ramp up in a month or two.

Quick Fit Plus: If you'd prefer a more demanding workout, gradually increase your speed to four miles per hour. Don't jog or run; just walk faster.

AEROBIC OPTION 1:
WALK ON THE TREADMILL

If you have access to a treadmill, I suggest you use it for Quick Fit, at least at the beginning. Set the treadmill for three miles per hour and walk for ten minutes—it's as simple as that.

If you've never used a treadmill before, please read pages 91–92 of Chapter 5; it will help you get started. If you're familiar with treadmills, you still might want to skim those pages, because they contain safety information.

AEROBIC OPTION 2:
WALK OUTDOORS

Most of my day is spent inside, so I appreciate the opportunity to step out. Fresh air is so energizing. Being outdoors gives me a whole different perspective, and I love it: I observe the change of seasons; I catch up with developments in the neighborhood. Give outdoor walking a try, even if you usually exercise indoors—you may become a convert.

For Quick Fit, you'll walk at three miles per hour. That's a brisk pace, not a stroll in the park where you stop to smell the roses. It's also not a walk with your dog, who stops at every tree. Walk the way you do when you know where you're going, you have an important appointment that starts in ten minutes, and you'll be late unless you step on it. One reason I suggest that you begin by doing Quick Fit on a treadmill, if possible, is that you'll learn from practice what three miles per hour feels like.

If you move at three miles per hour, a ten-minute walk covers half a mile. The simplest way to check your speed is to measure your route—which you need to do only once—and then wear a watch. You can measure the route by driving through it and keeping track on the car's odometer. Or you can use a pedometer (see Chapter 8, pages 173–174 for information about pedometers). If you live right near a track—or if you drop your kids off at school every day and can use the school track—that's a great place to walk. On a typical high school or college track, a lap is a quarter mile. So if you do two laps in ten minutes, you're on the right pace for Quick Fit. If it's an elementary or junior high school track, it may be shorter; call the school gym teacher and ask how long it is.

What about heat and cold, rain and snow? As they say in Norway, there's no such thing as bad weather, only bad clothing. Dress for comfort and relish the variety of outdoor walking—or have an indoor backup plan.

AEROBIC OPTION 3:
QUICK STEPS

Walking is a superb aerobic activity, but I realize that you may not have daily access to a treadmill or an appropriate outdoor walking route. That's where Quick Steps comes in. You can use Quick Steps as your daily aerobic activity, or you can do it occasionally instead of walking.

Quick Steps involves marching in place and five simple variations. All you need is a clear space about four feet by six feet. Foot-tapping music will make your workouts fun. Quick Steps is easy on your joints. There's no hopping or jumping; at least one foot remains on the floor at all times.

If you've ever taken a low-impact aerobics class, you'll be familiar with the variations—and if you haven't, you'll quickly learn them. Start with the leg moves, hands on hips. When you can do the steps automatically, add the arm movements to increase the intensity. If that makes the workout too strenuous, keep your hands on your hips and slow down if necessary.

One approach is to march in place for one minute, then do a variation for one minute. March again for a minute before switching to the second variation for one minute. And so on, until you've completed all five variations and ten minutes of aerobic activity. But feel free to improvise. You might want to march for the entire time; or you might prefer to use just one or two variations. And if you'd rather dance vigorously for ten minutes, that's fine, too.

Don't worry about "proper" form with Quick Steps—there isn't any! If you pass the song test (see page 108) and you're having a good time, you're doing it right.

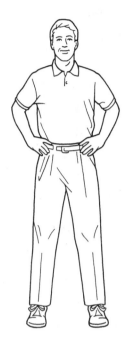

Marching in Place

Stand up tall. Put your hands on your hips. Start marching in place. When you walk, you land on your heel with each step. But when you march in place, your toe hits the ground first.

To Increase the Intensity

- Gradually increase the pace of your march.
- Raise your knees higher with each step.
- Pump your arms instead of keeping your hands on your hips.

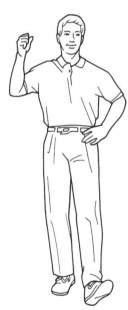

Variation 1: Front Heel Touch

- Stand up tall with your feet about six inches apart. Put your hands on your hips.
- Put your weight on your right foot.
- Move your left leg forward, bending your ankle so your toe points toward the ceiling. Touch your left heel to the floor.
- Bring your left foot back to its original position and step on it.
- Move your right leg forward and touch your right heel to the floor.
- Bring your right foot back to its original position and step on it.
- Repeat, alternating left and right heel touches.

To Increase the Intensity

- Pick up the pace and move more vigorously.
- Add arm movements: Imitate a hitchhiker. Make fists, with your thumb up. As your left leg goes forward, bring your left arm back and move your right arm up so that your thumb points toward your shoulder. Then, as your right leg goes forward, bring the right arm back and the left arm up in front.

Variation 2: Back Toe Touch

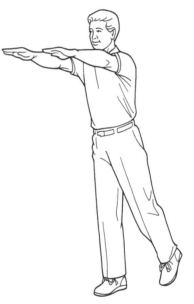

- Stand up tall with your feet about six inches apart. Put your hands on your hips.
- Put your weight on your right foot.
- Move your left leg back, pointing your toe toward the floor. Touch your left toe to the floor in back of you.
- Bring your left foot back to its original position and step on it.
- Move your right leg back and touch your right toe to the floor in back of you.
- Bring your right foot back to its original position and step on it.
- Repeat, alternating left and right touches. You may find it helpful to bend your knees and lean slightly forward with each toe touch.

To Increase the Intensity

- Pick up the pace or move more vigorously.
- Add arm movements: As you touch each toe, raise both arms straight in front of you. The higher your arms move, the more strenuous the workout.

Variation 3: Side Touch

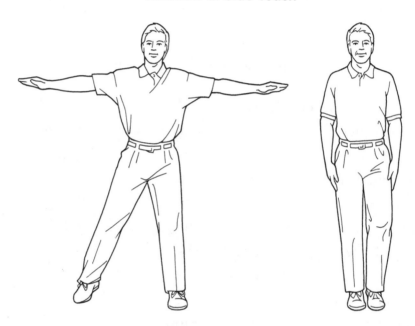

- Stand up tall with your feet together. Put your hands on your hips.
- Step to the right with your right foot. Your weight will be on the right foot. That was a side-step.
- Bring your left foot next to the right foot, but instead of stepping on the left foot, simply tap it. That was a touch.
- From the touch position, step to the left with your left foot.

Your weight is now on your left foot, and you've done another side-step.

- Bring your right foot next to the left and touch it.
- Repeat: Right side-step, left touch; left side-step, right touch.

To Increase the Intensity

- Pick up the pace.
- Move more vigorously: Take wider steps, bending your knees more.
- Add arm movements: As you step, move your arms out from your sides; as you touch, bring them back to your sides. For a more intense workout, raise your arms so that they're in line with your shoulders. If that leaves you breathless, raise them only halfway to shoulder height.

Variation 4: Front Kick

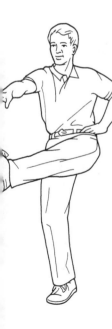

- Stand up tall with your feet about six inches apart. Put your hands on your hips.
- Put your weight on your right foot.
- Lift your left knee and kick your left leg forward, Rockette style.
- Step onto your left foot.
- Lift your right knee and kick your right leg forward.
- Repeat, alternating left and right kicks.

To Increase the Intensity

- Pick up the pace.
- Move more vigorously: Lift your knees higher and kick higher.
- Add arm movements: As you kick each leg, stretch the opposite arm out toward it. To make the arm movement more vigorous, raise your arms higher.

Variation 5: Hamstring Curl

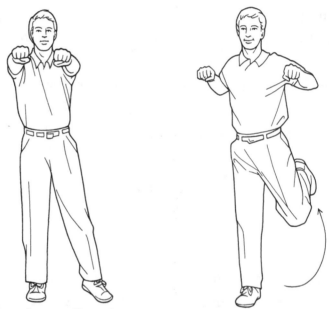

- Stand up tall with your feet about six inches apart. Put your hands on your hips.
- Put your weight on your right foot.
- Bend your left knee so that your left heel comes up in back of your body, as if you were trying to touch your rear end with your heel. That's a hamstring curl.

- Step onto your left foot.
- Bend your right knee and bring your right heel up in back of your body.
- Repeat, alternating left and right hamstring curls.

To Increase the Intensity

- Pick up the pace
- Move more vigorously, bending your knees as you step and lifting your heels higher with each hamstring curl.
- Add arm movements: With each step, move both arms straight in front of you, as if you were holding oars. With each hamstring curl, pull both arms back, as if you were rowing a boat. The higher you raise your arms and the harder you pull, the more strenuous the movement will be.

You've done ten minutes of aerobic activity—that's great! Your heart is beating faster but not pounding. You feel warm, but you're not sweating. You're two-thirds of the way through your Quick Fit workout, and you still have plenty of energy.

Next, you'll do four strengthening moves, one for your abs and three for your upper body. But first, I want to tell you about a bonus that I haven't mentioned before.

THE BONUS

In the process of doing the four strengthening exercises and the two stretches, you'll get up and down from the floor three times. Isn't that great?

When I'm teaching people about Quick Fit, I always hope they'll be delighted by this bonus. Instead, I usually hear groans from folks who haven't been on the floor since the 1960s when they took part in a college sit-in. Or someone will ask, "Wouldn't it be more efficient to do all the floor exercises at once, rather than getting down and up three times?"

"Sure," I reply, "it would be more efficient—but that's not what we're trying to accomplish here. It's efficient to drive half a mile to the store instead of walking; it's efficient to use a power lawn mower instead of the kind you push. You could run your whole household with a remote control, and you'd be so efficient that when you finally stood up, your weakened leg muscles would collapse under you!"

Let's get serious: I put the exercises in this order deliberately. Each time you get down and up again, you work the muscles in your legs, your abdomen, your back, and your arms, too, if you use them to assist. It really is a bonus for your workout. And think how important this ability becomes later in life. Sometimes seniors have to move out of their own homes or wear emergency call buttons ("I've fallen and I can't get up!"), simply because they're too weak to rise from the floor.

IS FLOOR EXERCISE A CHALLENGE?

- Do you have osteoporosis or any other physical condition that might make it risky for you to get down on the floor?
- Do you have problems with balance?
- Do you ever become faint when you sit up after you've been lying down, or when you stand after you've been sitting?
- Are you concerned about exercising on the floor for any reason—for example, are you worried about falling or fearful that once you're down you won't be able to get up?

If you answered "Yes" to any of these questions, talk with your doctor before doing any floor exercises. If you get a go-ahead, make sure that help is available in case you need assistance—especially when you're first starting Quick Fit. See pages 205–206 for a technique that uses a chair to assist.

If you can't get on the floor at all, do the floor exercises on your bed. (See pages 206–207 for more about that.) If you can get to the floor once, but three times would be too difficult, do all the standing exercises first. Then do all three floor exercises at the end of your workout, finishing with the Sit and Reach stretch.

As you become stronger, floor exercise may become feasible. Or you may be able to graduate from getting down once to getting down twice or even three times.

PART 2: MIDSECTION STRENGTH

1 MINUTE

The number one question people ask me about exercise is: "How can I get rid of *this*?" And they point to their belly. I always tell them: "You don't want to get rid of it; you just want to change the shape."

Toned abdominal muscles, sometimes called the abs, can improve your profile. But strong abs aren't just about how you look in a bathing suit. These muscles support our internal organs and our spine, and they help stabilize the body as we move.

The Abdominal Muscles

We have four abdominal muscles. Think of them as straps that go up and down and across our midsection, keeping the stomach, the liver, and the intestines properly stacked up on top of one another.

The rectus abdominis is a long, flat muscle that lies vertically in front of the torso. You contract this muscle when you bend forward. It's divided into two strips; in most people, each strip is subdivided into three sections. When the rectus abdominis is strengthened, these six sections form what's sometimes described as a "six-pack" or "washboard abs." Some highly trained athletes actually develop an eight-pack.

When you tie a package, you crisscross the rope to secure the contents. Similarly, you have two sets of abdominal muscles that run diagonally across the body, but in different directions. The external obliques form a V, starting with the pubic bone in the center, and going up to the ribs on both sides. Under the external obliques, and complementing them, are the internal obliques, which form an upside-down V. The internal and external obliques work together when you turn or bend to the side.

The last of the four abdominal muscles is the transversus abdominis, which lies under the rectus abdominis. As the name indicates, it runs horizontally across your midsection. Whenever you cough, sneeze, or breathe forcefully, this muscle contracts.

If our abdominal muscles go slack, our stacked-up internal organs shift. We can develop a paunch even if we haven't gained weight. Moreover, our back muscles must struggle to compensate. These problems improve as our abs become stronger. I can't tell you how many people come to me, puzzled, after a few months on Quick Fit and say, "Rick, I don't know what it is, but I've stopped getting backaches." They're surprised to learn that the same exercise that's flattening their abdomen is also helping their back.

Losing the Flab

Will Quick Fit give you a six-pack? Maybe. Will you actually be able to see the six-pack? Well, that depends. Strengthening exercise can firm and tone the muscles in your midsection. However, those magnificent muscles will be invisible if they're covered by a blanket of fat. A million crunches won't melt away abdominal fat. To get rid of it, you must lose weight.

That means burning calories with aerobic exercise and cutting back on excess food intake. Remember my motto: *Move a little more; eat a little less.* The more muscle you have, the easier this will be, because muscles burn more calories than fat.

Exercise for the Abs

When I was in college, the standard ab exercise was the sit-up. You lay flat on the floor, then you heaved yourself into a sitting position. There were two problems with these old-time sit-ups: First, they were hard on the back. Second, much of the effort didn't go into the abs, because part of the work was done by the leg and hip muscles—especially if you hooked your toes under a chair as you performed the move.

Today's ab exercises do a better job of protecting the back and focusing on the abdominal muscles. What about those expensive ab machines sold on TV? (See pages 209–210.) Not necessary. You don't need fancy equipment to tone your abs. In fact, one of the simplest ways to exercise your abdominal muscles is to pull your stomach in and hold it. I recommend this all the time. But when I look around, I see a lot of people who are not doing this exercise!

ABDOMINAL CRUNCH

Quick Fit's Abdominal Crunch will strengthen all your abdominal muscles. And there's a fitness extra: Because the move is done with your hands in front of your body, your neck muscles—which keep your head in position—get a workout, too. Stronger neck muscles improve posture and counter neck pain related to weak or fatigued muscles.

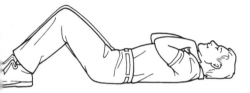 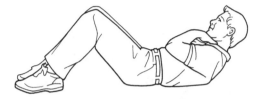

Starting Position

- Lie on your back on the floor.
- Bend your knees and place your feet flat on the floor, with your heels one to two feet away from your buttocks.
- Tilt your pelvis up slightly, so that the small of your back presses against the floor.
- Spread your thumbs and index fingers apart to make a V with each hand.
- Bring both hands up to the front of your neck, palms down, with one palm resting on the back of the other hand. No, you aren't going to choke yourself! Your hands become a chin rest in front of your neck. Gently touch your chin against the top hand and hold that position.

The Move

- Contract your abdominal muscles to pull your upper body up. Focus on crunching your abs. Your shoulders will move just three to six inches off the floor, no more.

- Release the contraction and return to the starting position.

Repetitions

- Do one set of ten crunches.
- Lie flat on the floor and relax for a few seconds.
- Resume the starting position and perform another set of ten crunches.

Form Check

✔ Does the small of your back remain on the floor throughout the exercise?

✔ Are you working your abs? One way to find out is to place this book on your abdomen. As you perform the crunches, the book should move up and down. Or you can place one hand on your abdomen to feel the muscle contract.

What to Watch Out For

Don't move up so far that the small of your back leaves the ground. That could strain muscles in your neck and lower back. You don't have to come up more than a few inches to give your abs a great workout.

The most common mistake I see in the gym is for someone to do this exercise with both hands behind his head, pushing his head forward with his hands. First, he could overextend his neck. Second, if he's just bobbing his head forward with each repetition, he's not working his abs by using them to lift his shoulders and head off the floor.

IF YOUR HEAD NEEDS SUPPORT

If your neck muscles currently are too weak to hold your head in position for the Abdominal Crunch, put one hand—not two!—behind your head for support. But don't use that hand to push the head forward. Keeping your other hand in front, serving as a chin rest, helps prevent that problem.

Because it's desirable to strengthen your neck muscles, work toward doing the Abdominal Crunches with both hands in front: Begin the exercise with both hands in front, if possible; support the neck only when it becomes necessary. As your neck muscles become stronger, the need for extra support should gradually disappear.

Customizing

Quick Fit Lite: If you can't manage two sets of ten crunches, do one set—or even part of one set—at first. But as your abdominal muscles become stronger, try adding one crunch to your workout. If that's not a strain, add another the next day. Add another the day after that, if you're able. And so on, until you're doing two sets of ten repetitions.

Quick Fit Plus: Gradually add crunches, working up to as many as fifty crunches in one minute. I recommend adding one crunch per day. At that rate, you can increase from two sets of ten to a total of fifty crunches in just one month. If you experience muscle soreness, cut back for a few days and then advance more slowly next time.

PART 3: UPPER BODY STRENGTHENING EXERCISES

3 MINUTES

The stronger you become, the easier your everyday activities will be. That's what fitness is all about. The next three exercises take a total of just three minutes. But in that short time, you'll strengthen your forearms and wrists, your biceps and triceps (the muscles in front and back of your upper arms), your shoulders, your lats (the latissimus dorsi, the fan-shaped back muscles that run under your arms), your chest, and your upper, middle, and lower back. What's more, your abdominal muscles get into the act, too, since they stabilize your body during the exercise. How's that for efficiency?

The three strengthening exercises require a pair of light dumbbells. (See pages 92–94 for information on dumbbells.) Because they're light, you won't feel the burn during your workout; you won't need ice packs the next day. But over time, your muscles will become stronger, firmer, and more toned.

To keep things simple, I suggest you use the same dumb-bells for all three exercises. Most women will use a pair of three-pound dumbbells to start; most men will use five-pound dumbbells. (See page 92 for instructions on selecting the starting weight that's right for you.) As you become stronger, you may want to swap your first pair of dumbbells for a heavier set (see pages 158–159 for more about this).

WHAT ABOUT BREATHING?

When I'm asked how to breathe during Quick Fit's strengthen-ing exercises, I usually say: "Don't worry about breathing—I promise you will do it!"

People who lift heavy weights need to pay attention to their breathing, because their blood pressure could spike if they hold their breath. But this precaution isn't necessary with the light weights you use for Quick Fit.

Nevertheless, if you think you might one day try a chal-lenging strength training program, why not get into good breathing habits. It's simple:

- Inhale before you start.
- Exhale as you lift the weight.
- Inhale again as you return to the starting position.

Some people like to focus on their breathing, even if the weights are light. This takes their mind off everyday matters and makes exercise almost like meditation. But most men and women who do Quick Fit prefer to keep things simple. One very easy and natural way to avoid holding your breath is to count out loud as you do the exercise. Even a whisper will do the trick.

Quick Fit Lite: If three-pound weights are too heavy, do the moves with one-pound weights (one-pound cans from the kitchen cupboard are okay, provided you can hold them securely). And if that's too hard, go through the exercises with no weights. Just lifting your arms will give you a workout if you're not yet strong. When this becomes easy, try one-pound weights. Then switch to three-pound dumbbells when you're ready.

Quick Fit Plus: If five-pound dumbbells are too light, use heavier weights. Increase the challenge gradually. Since you're doing Quick Fit every day, your muscles may become sore if the weights are too heavy.

BICEPS CURL

This move tones your wrists and forearms, as well as the biceps, those hardworking muscles in front of your upper arms. Everything you lift—whether it's a briefcase or a grocery bag—will feel lighter as these muscles become stronger.

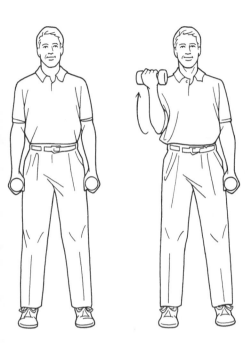

Starting Position

- Stand up tall—back straight, chest up, stomach in—with your feet flat on the floor and shoulder-width apart. There should be a slight bend in your knees, so you're comfortable and well balanced.
- Grasp the dumbbells firmly, holding one in each hand. Start with both arms at your sides, the palms parallel and facing your thighs.

The Move

- Only your forearms move during this exercise. Keeping your elbows at your sides, bend your right elbow to bring the dumbbell up.
- As you raise the dumbbell, turn your wrist so that your thumb points away from your body.
- Continue the move until the dumbbell is at shoulder level, with your palm facing your shoulder.
- Unbend your elbow to lower the dumbbell. Rotate your wrist so that your thumb points forward again. Keep your elbow against your side throughout the curl.
- At the end of the move, your arm should be back in the

starting position: At your side, fully extended, with your palm facing your thigh.

- Perform the same curl with your left arm.

Repetitions

Repeat, alternating right and left arms, until you have completed ten curls with each arm.

Form Check

✔ Are you standing tall, with knees slightly bent?
✔ Are both elbows at your sides throughout the curl?
✔ Is the move smooth and controlled?

What to Watch Out For

The most common mistake with this exercise is to swing the weights, letting them drop instead of lowering them in a controlled, deliberate way. This is not a good idea, for two reasons. First, you could hurt yourself. Second, if you allow gravity to do the work, your muscles won't benefit from the exercise.

Another problem I see frequently—especially when people attempt to use weights that are too heavy—is poor posture. Instead of standing tall, their hips are thrust forward, which puts strain on their upper and lower back.

FLOOR BENCH PRESS

This move strengthens three essential muscle groups: The pecs (the pectoralis major, your chest muscles), the shoulder muscles, and the triceps (the muscles in back of your upper arms). You use these muscles constantly: When you're typing on your computer, turning a steering wheel, or changing an overhead lightbulb.

Starting Position

This exercise is performed while you're lying on the floor (or on a bed if you can't get down on the floor).

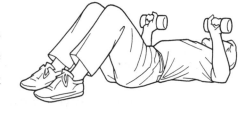

- Place the weights on the floor, positioning them so they'll be near your waist, one on your left and one on your right, when you're lying down.

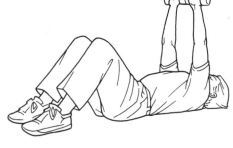

- Get down on the floor. Lie on your back. Bend your knees and place your feet flat on the floor, with your heels a foot or two away from your buttocks—the same position you used for the abdominal crunches.
- Grasp the dumbbells firmly, holding one in each hand. Lift

them by bending your elbows, as if you were doing biceps curls, until your forearms are perpendicular to the floor and your palms face each other.

- Slide your elbows on the floor, moving them away from your body, until your upper arms form a straight line with your shoulders. You're now in the starting position: Your upper arms are flat on the floor; your elbows are bent; your forearms are perpendicular to the floor; your wrists are straight. You are holding one dumbbell in each hand with your palms facing your feet.

The Move

- Push the dumbbells up toward the ceiling and toward each other. Extend your arms fully, but do not lock your elbows.
- Touch the ends of the dumbbells together *gently*, as if they were expensive crystal champagne glasses. This soft touch helps you remember to perform the move slowly and in a controlled way. The clink of the dumbbells is a toast to your good health.
- Lower the dumbbells to the starting position.

Repetitions

Repeat ten times. Then slide your elbows back to your sides, keeping your upper arms on the floor. Unbend your elbows to lower the weights.

Form Check

✔ Are your upper arms in a straight line with your shoulders?

✔ Are your wrists straight?

✔ As the dumbbells gently touch at the top of the lift, are your arms fully extended, with just a slight bend in your elbows?

What to Watch Out For

As you reach for the ceiling, it's tempting to reach a little too far and lock your elbows. But that puts pressure on your elbow joint, which could result in swelling and discomfort.

A common mistake with this exercise is to lower the dumbbells too quickly, letting gravity do the work. Some people bang their elbows on the floor, rather than lowering them in a controlled way. That could hurt your elbows (or annoy your downstairs neighbors!).

IF IT'S DIFFICULT TO LIE FLAT ON THE FLOOR

When some people try to lie flat on their back, they find that their head remains off the floor, which may be uncomfortable. If that happens to you when you do Quick Fit floor exercises, you can put a pillow under your head for support. But as you become more flexible, see if you can switch to a smaller pillow and eventually use no pillow at all. This will help you increase the range of motion in your neck and possibly improve your posture.

STANDING ROW

This simple move—like rowing, but done vertically—is specifically for the shoulders. Your shoulders participate in just about every activity that requires upper body motion, from setting the dinner table to chopping wood. Any time your arm is stretched out, your shoulder muscles are working. The tendons that connect the shoulder muscles to the bones are vulnerable. When you strengthen your shoulder muscles, you help prevent injury to the tendons.

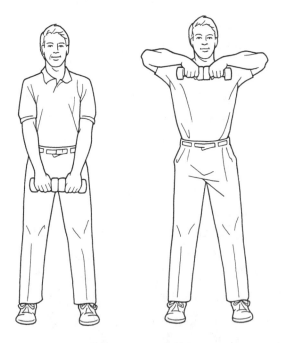

Starting Position

- Take the same position you took for the biceps curls: Stand up tall—back straight, chest up, stomach in—with your feet flat on the floor and shoulder-width apart. There should be a slight bend in your knees.

- Grasp the dumbbells firmly, holding one in each hand. Your arms should be down, fully extended. Your palms and the dumbbells should face the front of your body. Move your arms toward each other until the ends of the dumbbells lightly touch. That is the starting position.

The Move

- Pull the dumbbells straight up along the front of your body until they reach the top of your chest under your chin. Keep the ends of the dumbbells together throughout the move. This assures that both arms are moving together and in a controlled way.
- Your elbows will bend as you raise the dumbbells. Bend your wrists so that the dumbbells remain parallel to the floor as you lift them.
- At the end of the lift, the dumbbells will be just under your chin, parallel to the floor. Your elbows will be straight out to your sides, at shoulder height. Your upper arms and forearms will be parallel to the floor.
- Lower the dumbbells straight down along your body, keeping the ends touching each other, until you return to the starting position.

Repetitions

Repeat ten times.

Form Check

✔ Are you standing tall, with a slight bend in your knees?
✔ Do the ends of the dumbbells touch throughout the move?
✔ Are you maintaining control as you lower the dumbbells, rather than letting them drop?

What to Watch Out For

Bad posture is the most common mistake with this exercise. Stand up straight. Don't bend forward or hunch your shoulders as you lift the weights.

PART 4: STRETCHES | *1 MINUTE*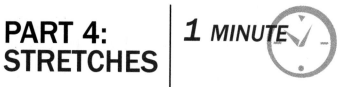

Quick Fit calls for one minute of stretching. You'll do two stretches: One for the upper body and one for the lower body. I sometimes do these stretches just before I go to bed, as well as after my workout, because I find that a nighttime stretch makes me more limber when I first wake up in the morning.

If you haven't stretched since high school gym class, you may be puzzled that stretching comes at the end of the workout rather than at the very beginning. That's because we now know from research that muscles gain the most benefit if they're warm when they're stretched.

SIDE BEND

This is the very best stretch I know of for the upper body—and it feels so good. You'll reach for the ceiling, which stretches muscles in your upper arms, your shoulders, your chest, and your upper back. At the same time, you'll bend to the side. That stretches the muscles in your middle and lower back, as well as your abdominal, groin, and inner thigh muscles.

The side bend is a dynamic stretch, which means that it's done while you're moving. Movement makes it easier for you to fully stretch to both sides of your body. You may have seen cautions against ballistic stretching, which also involves motion. However, that term usually refers to bouncing stretches that use momentum to push the body beyond its natural range of motion, which can cause injury. Dynamic stretches are safe because they involve gentle, controlled movement.

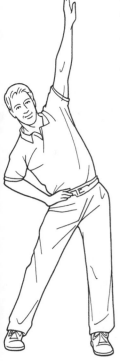

Starting Position

- Stand up tall—back straight, chest up, stomach in—with your feet flat on the floor and shoulder-width apart. There should be a slight bend in your knees.
- Put your hands on your hips.

The Move

- Lift your left arm straight up over your head, reaching for the ceiling. Simultaneously, bend to your right side. Your left arm continues to reach straight up; it does not arch over your head, because that position would not allow it to stretch. Keep both feet flat on the floor throughout the stretch.
- Return to the starting position, standing tall with both hands on your hips.
- Repeat on the other side, keeping both feet flat on the floor throughout the move: Bend to your left side, simultaneously lifting your right arm up to the ceiling; then return to the starting position.

Repetitions

Repeat the side bends, alternating sides, for thirty seconds. During this time you should complete approximately ten bends to each side. You can count bends or watch the clock, as you prefer.

Where You'll Feel the Stretch

You'll feel the stretch through your upper arms, shoulders, and back, as well as in your waist, abdomen, inner thigh, and groin.

Form Check

✔ Are your feet flat on the floor throughout the stretch, knees slightly bent?

✔ Are you bending side to side only, and not bending forward?

✔ Does your arm reach straight up, rather than curling over your head like a halo?

What to Watch Out For

Don't move too quickly, and don't bounce—that leads to over-stretching, which could be painful. Stretches should be gentle and controlled.

Customizing

Quick Fit Lite: If you can't reach up so your hand points toward the ceiling, reach up as far as you can. Similarly, bend only slightly to the side, if that's all you can manage. Move more slowly, doing fewer side bends if necessary. As you become more flexible, you'll be able to reach and bend farther.

Quick Fit Plus: Extend your range of motion by bending farther to the side. But keep it gentle and never stretch to the point of pain.

SIT AND REACH

This is my favorite stretch, because it allows you to relax totally. You don't have to contract a single muscle; you don't have to stand erect. In just thirty seconds, you stretch muscles and tendons along the full length of your body: The bottoms of your feet, your ankles, the Achilles tendons in back of your ankles, your calf muscles, the muscles and tendons behind your knees, the hamstring muscles in back of your thighs, the muscles in your buttocks and lower, middle, and upper back, your shoulder muscles, and the muscles in the back of your neck. Wow!

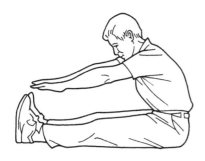

Starting Position

Sit on the floor with your legs together and straight out in front of you. There should be a slight bend in your knees. Point your toes toward the ceiling.

The Move

- Reach your arms toward your toes and lean forward until you feel the pull of the stretch, but no pain. Depending on your flexibility, you may reach your thighs, your knees, your shins, or your toes. (See below for Quick Fit Lite if you can't reach your thighs.)
- If you can, grasp the tips of your toes so you don't need

your muscles to hold you in position. If you can't reach that far, lean forward and place your hands on top of your thighs, knees, or shins. Let your head bend forward, but don't overextend your neck; your chin should not touch your chest.

- Relax and enjoy the stretch.

Hold

Hold the stretch for thirty seconds.

Where You'll Feel the Stretch

You'll feel the stretch through the bottoms of your feet, your ankles, the backs of your legs, your back, shoulders, and neck.

Form Check

✔ Is there a slight bend in your knees?
✔ Are your toes pointed up toward the ceiling?
✔ Is your chin away from your chest?

What to Watch Out For

People sometimes bob and bounce when they do this exercise, struggling to touch their toes. But that can cause painful overstretching. Flexibility varies from individual to individual. Your full range of motion may not include touching your toes—and that's fine. Just reach as far as you comfortably can. Over time, this stretch will help you maintain and even extend your range of motion.

Customizing

Quick Fit Lite: If you can't easily sit on the floor without support, sit with your back leaning against a wall. This alone will enable you to feel a stretch. If it's too difficult to sit against the wall, with your torso at a 90-degree angle to your legs, increase the angle by moving your rear end away from the wall. As you become more flexible, you'll be able to move closer to the wall, decreasing the angle between your torso and your legs. Eventually you may be able to do the regular Quick Fit version of this stretch, without the wall. Note: If you can't sit on the floor, do the same moves while sitting on a bed.

Quick Fit Plus: Extend your range of motion, gently bending as far forward as you can without pain. Always move in a slow, controlled manner, without bouncing.

Congratulations! You've completed your first Quick Fit workout. That's all there is to it! You've done ten minutes of aerobic exercise, to get your heart rate up. You've worked your abdominal muscles and the muscles in your upper body. And you've given yourself a good stretch from head to toe. Because you're just learning the program, you probably needed extra time. But once you're familiar with the workout—and that doesn't take long if you do it every day—you'll be done in fifteen minutes.

From your very first workout, you'll experience benefits: You'll be warmed up and energized, as well as loose and relaxed. Enjoy the feeling—and make Quick Fit part of your day, every day!

RICK BRADLEY'S
QUICK FIT IN A FLASH

PART 1: AEROBIC EXERCISE (10 MINUTES)

OPTION 1: Walk on the treadmill at three miles per hour

OPTION 2: Walk outdoors at three miles per hour

OPTION 3: Quick Steps

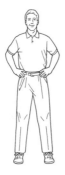 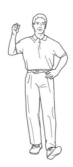 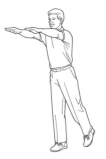

- MARCH
  (one minute)

- FRONT HEEL
  TOUCH
  (one minute)
- MARCH
  (one minute)

- BACK TOE TOUCH
  (one minute)
- MARCH
  (one minute)

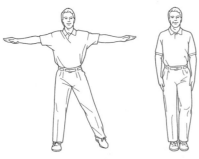 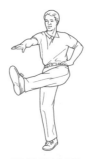 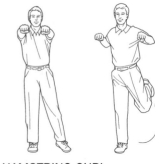

- SIDE TOUCH (one minute)
- MARCH (one minute)

- FRONT KICK
  (one minute)
- MARCH
  (one minute)

- HAMSTRING CURL
  (one minute)

144
from *Quick Fit: The Complete 15-Minute No-Sweat Workout*
by Richard Bradley III, with Sarah Wernick (Atria Books, 2004)

PART 2: ABDOMINAL STRENGTHENING EXERCISE (1 MINUTE)

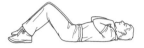 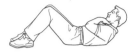

• ABDOMINAL CRUNCH (two sets of ten repetitions)

PART 3: UPPER BODY STRENGTHENING EXERCISES (3 MINUTES)

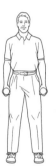 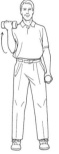 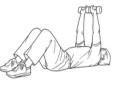 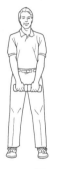 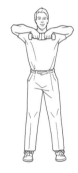

BICEPS CURL (ten repetitions with each arm)

• FLOOR BENCH PRESS (ten repetitions)

• STANDING ROW (ten repetitions)

PART 4: STRETCHES (1 MINUTE)

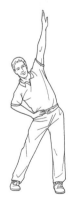 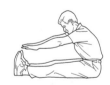

• SIDE BEND (thirty seconds or ten bends to each side)

• SIT AND REACH (thirty seconds)

A MOTIVATIONAL PLAN

You've made the commitment to start Quick Fit; you've learned the moves. Now you know how easy and simple this program is. Success with Quick Fit does *not* require athletic ability! But it does require brain power. That's because every exercise regimen—even one that takes just fifteen minutes—needs a motivational plan. And a motivational plan takes some ingenuity.

What will you do to enable yourself to stick with this program, day after day? How will you make exercise as satisfying and enjoyable as possible? How will you handle the inevitable problems? This chapter offers many suggestions.

THINK POSITIVELY

Positive thinking works for everything in life. When you think positively, you become more motivated. Action follows naturally. It's as simple as that.

I realize that working out may not be your idea of a good time. Fortunately, you don't have to love exercise to get all the benefits. However, doing it consistently—day after day, month after month—will be a lot easier if you focus your attention on the positives. There really is a lot to like. You may surprise yourself and find that you actually look forward to your workouts.

Get Excited About the Benefits

Notice all the ways that exercise enhances your life. Everyone can expect improvements, big and small. But the less fit you were when you started, the more change you can expect.

More Energy and Stamina

Life is easier when you can take care of things without undue stress and strain. I hope you get a kick out of your increased vitality.

Improved Heart and Lung Power

When you climb a flight of stairs or run to catch a bus—and notice that you aren't puffing from the effort—give yourself a pat on the back. Daily aerobic activity is paying off. Nancy reported:

The other day I had to get home for an appointment and I had to run to catch the train. I was loaded down with a gym bag, a shopping bag, and my purse. I had to run down a long platform, up a flight of stairs, then down another flight of stairs, and down another platform. We're talking about a heroic effort here! I made the train. I was very happy to be able to run like that. Before Quick Fit, I could barely walk that distance.

Increased Strength

Quick Fit strengthens your entire body. Your upper body gets a workout from the weights, while the muscles in your lower body benefit both from walking and from getting down on the floor and up again three times a day. Your empowered muscles will surprise and delight you. Suddenly, yard work is no problem. Two grocery bags don't feel very heavy. You can carry a sleepy child and your arms don't ache.

In the last year or so I'd had trouble getting up from a squatting position when I was digging around for a pan in back of the lower cupboard. Not anymore. I see a significant improvement in my ability to get myself upright. I am working toward the day when I leap up, pan in hand.

—ANNE

A Trimmer Body

Over time, you may shed a few pounds, just because you're more active now. Even without changes in your weight, you may look slimmer. Enjoy what you see in the mirror. Your posture will be better. There will be less jiggle in your upper arms and in your neck. Your clothes may fit more loosely because your muscles are toned.

Janine wasn't trying to lose weight. But two months after starting Quick Fit, she discovered that she had dropped several pounds:

> *I'm blessed with a metabolism that responds well to exercise. After I lost weight, I tried on the fancy pants suit that I was going to wear to an awards banquet, and I was swimming in it. That wasn't a terrible problem—I'm happy to have a little muscle tone in my arms.*
>
> *I went shopping with a friend to buy a different outfit for the banquet. When I tried it on, and she saw how my arms looked, she said, "What is this exercise program? I want in on it."*

Greater Flexibility

If you had become resigned to feeling stiff in the morning, you may have a pleasant surprise after several months of daily stretching with Quick Fit. Appreciate your increased range of motion, whether you're reaching to scrub your back in the shower or stretching to retrieve something that's fallen behind a cabinet.

Long-Term Health Benefits

Health changes don't happen overnight. But at your annual checkup, you may find that high blood pressure and cholesterol numbers have dropped to healthy levels.

Notice How Good Exercise Makes You Feel

Our bodies were made to move. Once we become acclimated to exercise, it feels so good. Love those endorphins! Pay attention to the mood lift you get from aerobic activity. Feel tension melt away. Observe how your mind seems quicker after your workout. Savor the satisfaction of accomplishing something important for your health. Chuck, a member of our test group, said:

I think the greatest benefit is psychological—the feeling that I am doing something each day that is good for me physically.

Remember these terrific feelings. Make them part of your mental picture of Quick Fit. The more you associate your workout with positive experiences, the more motivated you will be.

———————————

One morning I woke up and my neck felt as if it was locked. A migraine was hovering. I dragged myself out of bed and tried to limber up by walking around the house. I took a hot shower and made coffee. I felt marginally better, but the migraine was still hovering. I wondered: Should I try to do Quick Fit? I didn't feel like it but told myself, "I'll at least start the walking part and see how it goes." I pulled on my shoes and went out.

I found myself thoroughly enjoying the walk. Looking at trees and flowers, walking along and swinging my arms, relaxed me and really loosened up my muscles. One of the bad things with chronic pain is that you tense against it. So ultimately you wind up with more pain because of your fear. When I finished my walk, I felt revived.

—Rowshana

Take Pride in Your Consistency

Thanks to Quick Fit, you're a New You! You used to be sedentary, and now you're a person who works out daily. Becoming consistent about exercise is a real accomplishment. Think about that and congratulate yourself after each workout.

MONITOR YOUR PROGRESS

At the DOT Fitness Center, some people write down the number of calories they burn in each exercise session. One man, who spends an hour each day on a very demanding routine, burns over 100,000 calories a year. Other people count the number of miles they walk. If they're on Quick Fit, they walk three and a half miles per week. Those numbers add up!

Quick Fit will improve your aerobic capacity and make you stronger and more flexible. However, this doesn't happen instantly. Because the changes are gradual, you might not notice them unless you pay attention. But if you keep track, you'll see how much progress you've made—which will motivate you to make more.

A Record of Consistency

In 1988, I began keeping a record of my daily workouts. This was a particularly hectic period for me. In addition to my demanding job at the U.S. Department of Transportation, I spent as much time as possible with my son, Ryan, who was then seven years old. Between Ryan's soccer practice, soccer games, basketball practice, and basketball games, I sometimes didn't have time for my own daily workouts.

I decided to keep track of my exercise for a month, something I'd never done before. I took a blank piece of paper and drew a grid with thirty-one boxes across for the days and five rows down, one for each of the exercises in my routine. Each evening I'd take a yellow marker and fill in the squares for the exercises I'd done that day. At the end of the month, that piece of paper looked like a checkerboard. As I stared at it, dismayed by all the white squares, I resolved to do better.

The next month my grid of days and exercises was solid yellow. In fact, the next time a white square appeared in my monthly workout chart was four years later, in 1992, when I was recovering from surgery. So I'm sold on the motivational power of records.

Some people enjoy keeping an exercise diary. But it's enough to make a tiny check on your calendar every day after your workout. At the end of each month, glance at your record.

- If you're doing Quick Fit just about every day, congratulations!
- If you usually miss one or two workouts per week, you're well on your way to establishing an exercise habit. But try to become more consistent.
- If you're missing more than two workouts per week, see pages 164–165 later in this chapter. Set yourself a goal for next week to do five workouts. When you're back on track, make daily exercise your goal.

Improved Aerobic Capacity

You'll see many improvements in everyday life after you've been doing Quick Fit for a while. You'll also see progress during exercise sessions. As you become fitter, your workouts will seem easier. Some people focus on these changes, because they find them encouraging. Others decide to challenge themselves to work harder, and they draw encouragement from their progress. Take whatever approach is best for you.

Gradually Increase Exercise Intensity

When you started Quick Fit (unless you opted for Quick Fit Lite or Plus), you walked at three miles per hour or did the equivalent with Quick Steps. After a few weeks or months, depending on your age and previous fitness level, your heart and lungs adjust to that pace. You probably could go faster without undue strain. As long as you still pass the song test (see page 108), you're not working too hard.

If you're using a treadmill, increase the speed by one-tenth of a mile per hour (.1 mph). See how that feels. Can you still sing one line of a song in a single breath? When you're accustomed to this slightly faster pace, try another one-tenth-of-a-mile-per-hour increase. If you like, work your way up to four miles per hour, a very brisk walk.

If you're doing Quick Steps, you can add intensity by moving more quickly or by adding arm movements. The higher you raise your arms, the more strenuous Quick Steps will be.

Follow Your Heart

As your heart becomes stronger, the same activity requires less effort. By monitoring your heart rate, you can see even small changes in fitness. Some people find this concrete evidence of improvement motivating. Those who prefer simplicity can skip this section.

If you're a typical adult, your heart beats approximately seventy to seventy-five times per minute when you're sitting quietly. This is called your resting heart rate. People who are out of shape tend to have higher resting heart rates. On the other hand, trained athletes, whose hearts become very efficient, typically have much lower resting heart rates. For example, Lance Armstrong, the champion cyclist, reportedly has a resting heart rate of only thirty-two beats per minute.

How fast can your heart beat—in other words, what's the maximum? Individuals vary, but in general, the answer depends more on age than upon fitness level. Typically, the maximum heart rate in childhood is about 220 beats per minute. But the number usually decreases by about one beat per minute per year, even for athletes.

You can estimate your maximum heart rate by subtracting your age in years from 220. For instance, if you're 30 years old, your maximum heart rate is about 190 beats per minute (220 minus 30); if you're 60, it's 160 beats per minute (220 minus 60).

Aerobic exercise should raise your heart rate, but not to the max. A reasonable goal for Quick Fit is to exercise at a level that keeps your heart rate at 50 to 75 percent of your estimated maximum. This range is your target heart rate. If you don't want to do the math, WebMD.com will perform the calculation at *http://my.webmd.com/heartrate*, if you fill in your age. Or use the table on the next page.

Age	Maximum Heart Rate (220 - age in years)	Target Heart Rate (50 to 75 percent of maximum)
20	200	100–150
25	195	98–146
30	190	95–143
35	185	93–139
40	180	90–135
45	175	88–131
50	170	85–128
55	165	83–124
60	160	80–120
65	155	78–116
70	150	75–113
75	145	73–109
80	140	70–105
85	135	68–101
90	130	65–98

All you need to measure your heart rate is a clock or watch with a second hand. Do the following right after you finish your aerobic activity, so you don't interrupt your workout:

• Put your hand on your chest or place your fingers on the pulse at your wrist and find the beat. If you can't locate it right away, keep looking—I guarantee you have a heartbeat!

- Using a clock or watch, count the number of beats in ten seconds.
- Multiply that number by six to get the beats-per-minute rate.

Are you in the target range for a person your age? If you're too low, increase your pace the next time; if you're too high, slow down.

Serious athletes use electronic heart rate monitors to get precise data. That's strictly optional for anyone doing Quick Fit. But if you love gadgets and numbers, you might find the information motivating.

A heart rate monitor consists of a belt with sensors, which you strap around your chest, and a device that looks like a wristwatch, which can receive signals from the belt. A basic model costs about $50; more elaborate versions— which can calculate workout statistics or beep to remind you to exercise—run $100 to $200 or even more.

If you work out at a health club, ask if they have a treadmill with sensors on the handrail that can measure your heart rate. Also, some treadmills can receive signals from heart rate monitor belts and display the numbers, so you don't have to use the wrist device.

Greater Strength

Many people who do Quick Fit are content to stick with the three- or five-pound weights they used when they started the program. But you'll get stronger, and you'll be more aware of your progress, if you move up.

If you decide to increase the weight, here's how to tell if it's time for a change: Ask yourself how your arms feel when you finish the three strengthening exercises.

- If you think you could keep going all day, the weights are too light.
- If your muscles ache from the effort, the weights are too heavy.
- If you're comfortable and you know you could continue for a while if you needed to, but the dumbbells feel heavier now than they did when you started—the weights are about right.

To avoid muscle soreness, progress gradually. Use a pair of dumbbells for at least two weeks before you graduate to heavier ones. I suggest a maximum of fifteen pounds per dumbbell for men (that's what I use) and ten pounds per dumbbell for women. You may have friends who lift much heavier weights. But when people use heavy weights that bring their muscles to fatigue, they need a day of rest between workouts. Since Quick Fit is done daily, lighter weights are called for.

Improved Flexibility

Your daily Quick Fit stretches will make you more flexible. That means less fatigue and fewer aches and pains. When your body is stiff, you fight with yourself every time you bend over to tie your shoes or reach up to get a book off the top shelf. Life is a lot easier when you're more flexible.

A simple way to chart your progress is to note how far you can reach during the Sit and Reach stretch.

- Can you do the exercise without leaning against a wall?
- Can you reach your knees? Your ankles? Your toes?
- Can you reach beyond your toes? By how much?

As you continue to do Quick Fit every day, you can expect improvements in your flexibility over time.

ADD VARIETY

Routines and habits keep you on track. But throw in a little variety to add interest and stay motivated.

Vary Your Aerobic Activity

Your heart doesn't care what you do for aerobic exercise. It just knows that you're doing *something* and that it needs to work harder to pump more oxygen.

- If you're walking outdoors, take a new route for a change of scene.
- If you haven't yet done Quick Steps (see pages 110–117), give that a try.

- If you're working out at a gym, switch occasionally from the treadmill to an elliptical walker, a rowing machine, or a stationary bike.
- Break your routine with swimming, bike riding, dancing, or other exerting activities.

Vary Your Entertainment

Many people divert themselves while doing Quick Fit. They may watch a favorite television program or listen to lively music. But after a while, the same entertainment becomes less of a treat. So switch occasionally. Try a new TV show or tape a rerun; buy yourself a new CD. Or come up with an entirely different diversion. Listen to a recorded book. Or do your workout with a friend once or twice a week.

LEARN TO DEAL WITH DISRUPTIONS

No matter how motivated and dedicated you are, your fitness routine will be disrupted from time to time. But fitness is a lifelong project. In the long run, the skipped sessions don't matter. What counts is that you get back on track.

If You're Unwell

When you're so sick that you can't get out of bed, you know you must skip your workout. But what if you're simply under the weather?

Ask yourself if you'll feel better or worse if you exercise. Sometimes exercise actually makes you feel better. For example, if you have a cold, aerobic activity may clear your stuffy nose temporarily. But if you have a throbbing headache, walking may make you feel worse. In that case, don't do it! If you aren't sure, give it a try for a minute or two and then decide whether to stop or continue.

If an illness forces you to take a break from Quick Fit, you may need to ease yourself back into your workouts. After three days of inactivity, your body begins to decondition. When you resume, you might need to use lighter weights, or to do regular Quick Fit instead of Quick Fit Plus. Please don't be discouraged by this temporary setback. If you gradually increase the intensity of your workouts, you'll soon return to full capacity.

When You're on the Road

Quick Fit can be done just about anywhere. Walking in a new environment is exciting—and it's a great way to find the best restaurants, sights, and shops. If you can't walk outdoors and a treadmill isn't available, do Quick Steps.

I traveled to attend festivities at my old high school. The days were chopped up, with a lot of meetings, luncheons, and tours. A couple of times I had to go to a shopping mall to pick something up. Instead of driving to the mall, I used the opportunity to walk. I felt noble!

—CHUCK

The abdominal curls and the stretches need no special equipment. But what about the exercises that require dumbbells? These days, many hotels have fitness facilities, or they can arrange for you to have a day pass to a nearby gym. Tina took a cruise to Tahiti about six weeks after she started Quick Fit. She not only kept up with her workouts on the ship, but she actually advanced:

The ship's spa had a treadmill and weights. I exercised every day. Before the trip I was using three-pound weights. But on the ship, the smallest weights they had were five pounds, so I used those!

Some people take their weights with them. But if you prefer to travel light, consider these two options:

- Exercise tubes are light, stretchy tubes that can be used for strengthening exercises. Look for a version that comes with handles; they're easier to hold without straining your wrists. An instructional booklet is also helpful. Price: $5 to $15.
- Inflatable plastic dumbbells, called AquaBells, are light to carry but become heavy when filled with water at your destination. These are sold by some sporting goods and travel

stores (for example, Fitness First, mentioned on page 93 in Chapter 5). Or contact AquaBells Travel Weights (800-987-6892; *http://www.aquabells.com*). Price: $50.

If You Stop or Can't Get Started

Your workouts may be disrupted by emergencies, work demands, family problems, obligations, other people's needs, mechanical breakdowns, bad weather, unexpected situations—in other words: Life. Welcome to the club! Now figure out how to get moving again.

If you can't seem to get started—or if you've begun but usually miss more than one or two sessions a week—something needs to change. Ask yourself a few questions:

- What's getting in the way? You might find it helpful to reread Chapter 3, which discusses the common obstacles to regular physical activity.
- Is Quick Fit on your To Do List? If you've been winging it—and it's not working—the time has come to schedule your workouts.
- Why do you want to exercise? In Chapter 4, before you got started, I suggested that you focus on all the reasons that you want to get fit. Think about them again. Many people have told me that writing down their motives to do Quick Fit really helped firm up their resolve.
- Give first-thing-in-the-morning workouts a try. The best way I know to guarantee consistency is to exercise early in

the day. Remember: Nothing can interfere with a completed workout.

For me, it's literally wake up, clean up, and in ten minutes I'm out the door for my walk. I don't eat, don't have coffee. This is the way I get going in the morning. I'm up early, so I often see a sunrise. For me, it's symbolically stimulating to see the change from darkness to light.

—ANTHONY

If you've fallen off track, simply pick yourself up and get started again. Don't try to catch up in one day. If you've stopped for several weeks, start from the beginning. You'll actually get up to speed more quickly if you don't overdo it.

CELEBRATE YOUR VICTORIES

When Fitness Center members tally up 100 miles I give them a T-shirt that says: "100 Mile Club." Now a T-shirt is not exactly a lavish reward. But it's still a motivator. I also give out baseball hats, water bottles, and key chains as little incentives.

The biggest prize I offer is the Fitness Consistency

Award—a beautiful jacket that says: "DOT Fitness Center." Every six months I give away one each to the man and woman who have visited the Fitness Center most consistently over the past six months. People have actually rescheduled their annual leave to win this award, which shows how powerful a reward can be.

I hope you'll figure out ways to celebrate your Quick Fit consistency milestones. You might treat yourself to a night out on the town, buy yourself something luxurious, or visit a day spa for a massage. Think of something that will motivate you.

Prizes and other material rewards are fun. But you can't buy the most important rewards of exercise: All the health benefits of becoming fit and—even more important—feeling good about yourself for keeping this commitment.

MOVING BEYOND QUICK FIT

You've been consistent with Quick Fit for several months, and it's made a difference. You feel terrific; you look good, too. You're solidly committed to the program. That's great! Just keep doing Quick Fit, every day.

However, some of you may be so enthusiastic that you want to become even more active. Excellent! This chapter offers many options for moving beyond Quick Fit. I'll suggest ways you can add other kinds of physical activity to your life. You'll also learn four new strengthening moves and two new stretches that complement the basic Quick Fit program. If you add those and also increase your aerobic activity, you could reach the goal set by the U.S. surgeon general: Half an hour of moderately intense physical activity on all or most days of the week. That would be quite an accomplishment. Less than one-third of Americans meet this standard.

WHY CHANGE A WINNER?

Many people tell me that Quick Fit is the first exercise program they've ever been able to stick with. The last thing they want to do is tinker with success. Pauline said:

I like the simplicity. I like the fact that I do it every single day. With Quick Fit, I know what I have to do, I do it—and then I get on with my life. It's not fancy. It doesn't require special clothing, I don't have to figure out complicated machinery. Quick Fit works for me. I'm content to do it for the rest of my life.

If you feel the same way, I wish you a long and healthy lifetime with Quick Fit. You'll gain many health benefits from doing this program every day.

But if you're interested in the possibility of moving beyond Quick Fit, I hope you'll explore the options described in this chapter. The more exercise you do, within reason, the more health benefits you can expect. Findings from the College Alumni Health Study (described in Chapter 2) suggest that someone who does Quick Fit—burning about 500 calories per week—enjoys a 27 percent reduction in mortality compared to those who aren't active at all. But the improvements in longevity are even better if you do more.

Expanding your workouts is also great for weight control. The more calories you burn, the easier it is to shed excess pounds and maintain a healthy weight. You'll like the way your new body looks, firmed and toned by strengthening exercise.

Remember, it's best to increase physical activity *gradually*, for two reasons. First, you allow your body to adjust to the new demands. Second, you give yourself time to incorporate new behavior into your lifestyle. If you do too much too quickly, you risk muscle soreness and burnout.

> *Consider Quick Fit your minimum daily requirement.*
> *You can always do more—*
> *but never less.*

MOVE A LITTLE MORE

Most men empty their pockets when they get undressed at night. Then the next morning, they put everything back. But one guy I know drops all the change—pennies, nickels, dimes, quarters, and the occasional half dollar—into a large bottle. Just before the end of the year, he spills out the contents and counts the coins. One year he collected more than $500, and it's never been less than $250. He and his wife use this "found" money to splurge on a weekend holiday.

In the same way, every minute of exercise counts. Over the sixteen hours of your waking day, all those minutes add up. And over a year, they can make a significant difference.

Exercise You Won't Notice

People who have been doing Quick Fit for a while often become more active without even thinking about it. They aren't doing longer workouts, they're just moving more than in the past. Instead of sliding behind the wheel to run an errand, they walk. Rather than waiting for the elevator, they climb the stairs.

You may have noticed this kind of spontaneous change. It's not surprising: Thanks to Quick Fit, you have more energy and stamina. You're also stronger and more flexible, so it's easier to move. Now think about increasing your everyday physical activity *deliberately*. Some possibilities:

- Look for opportunities to walk. Do you ever see people drive around a shopping center parking lot for five minutes, looking for a spot near the entrance, so they can spare themselves a three-minute walk? Park on the edge of the lot. You'll save time and clock some extra exercise. Forget about step-saving maneuvers, like placing the trash can right next to your desk. A little inefficiency makes you fitter.
- Use the free exercise machine in your home or office. I'm referring to the staircase. Also take the stairs in shopping centers or when you have a medical appointment. If you climb up and down a flight of stairs, you burn about 8 calories. Do this three times daily, and after a year that pocket change adds up to 8,760 calories, the equivalent of about two and a half pounds.

I take the stairs instead of elevators. It gives me a sense of achievement: At sixty-seven I'm still young enough to climb four flights of stairs. I don't have to creep up; it doesn't hurt—and I don't get winded!

—*CHUCK*

- Don't just sit there; stand up and move. If you watch TV, march in place or do Quick Steps during the commercials. After a one-hour show, you will have moved for about twelve minutes. Keep this up for a week, and you'll accumulate nearly one and a half hours of extra exercise. If you're talking on the phone, walk around the room.

- If you're getting together with a friend or colleague, suggest meeting for a walk rather than for drinks, coffee, or lunch.

- Use the wrong hand. If you're right-handed, use your left hand to push the vacuum cleaner or play tennis; lefties, switch to the right. You'll use more energy that way, because you're less efficient when you work with your nondominant hand.

- Don't waste waiting time. Walk in place or do Quick Steps when you're standing in line or waiting for a bus or train. If you commute to work, and your average wait is three minutes in each direction, that's thirty extra minutes of physical activity every week.

- Squirm. Cross and uncross your legs. Bounce in your chair. Scientists at the Mayo Clinic found that some people burn nearly 700 calories a day this way. The scientists call it "nonexercise activity thermogenesis." My wife calls it fidgeting.

- Make life a little less convenient. Some experts blame the obesity epidemic on modern labor-saving gadgets—everything from washing machines to TV remotes. Do things the old-fashioned way. Oil up the push-it-yourself lawn mower. Walk to the pizza shop instead of dialing or clicking for takeout.

This "lifestyle exercise"—extra walking, stair climbing, and active chores like gardening—can be just as effective as strenuous workouts at the gym, according to a study from the Cooper Institute for Aerobics Research.

Investigators recruited 235 sedentary men and women and assigned them at random to two groups. One group followed a traditional exercise program; the other simply added thirty minutes of lifestyle exercise to their day. After six months, the two groups showed similar improvements in fitness, as well as similarly lowered numbers for blood pressure, cholesterol, and body fat.

POSTURE PICKUP

Here's a one-minute ab exercise that can be done anytime, anyplace. Stand up tall, with your back straight and your head up, so that the bottom of your chin is parallel to the floor. Now tighten your abdominal muscles. That's all there is to it: Just suck in your gut and hold it for one minute. You'll improve your posture while giving your abdominal muscles a mini workout.

Does this sound familiar? Yes, it's the position you take for the Biceps Curl and Standing Row. When you do those exercises, you're also working your abs—yet another Quick Fit bonus.

Count Your Steps

How many steps do you take every day? That includes everything, from going to the bathroom after you wake up in the morning, to visiting a colleague down the hall, to walking around the kitchen as you prepare dinner and set the table.

If you work at a desk and your main leisure activity is reading or watching TV, you might take 1,000 or even fewer steps per day. The average American does a little better, maybe 2,000 to 5,000 steps a day. But if you can manage to accumulate 10,000 steps per day, you'd actually meet the U.S. surgeon general's exercise guidelines.

Walking is a great way to tuck extra activity into your life. If you clip a pedometer to your waistband, you can keep track of your steps. Everyone I know who has tried it says that the numbers are a terrific motivator. You can pick up a pedometer in any sporting goods store, or you can order one online or by phone (see resource list on page 93). Expect to pay about $15 to $25 for a basic model that simply counts your steps; that's all you need. Fancier versions give you calorie counts and other extra information.

Here's a simple and gradual way to increase the amount of walking you do, with the help of a pedometer:

- Wear a pedometer for a week, without making a special effort to walk more. Put it on when you get dressed in the morning. Take it off when you get undressed at night. Keep a pad by your bed and jot down your total steps at the end of every day.

- After a week, check your daily record of steps. Circle the highest number. That's your goal for next week. Note: If you walked an exceptional amount on one day, take the next highest number. The idea is to push your limits, but gently.

- During the second week, continue to wear the pedometer and to record your steps. Try to meet your goal every day. Look for easy, natural opportunities to walk more, like using a less convenient bathroom or telephone at home or work. At the end of the week, look at the numbers again, circle the highest one, and come up with a new goal.

- Continue to set a new, slightly higher goal each week. Try to develop habits that encourage walking, such as taking a longer route when you go to the post office or library. Seeing your success in the pedometer readings will be very encouraging.

ADD OTHER EXERCISE

Quick Fit is a gateway exercise: It opens the door to other physical activities. You will feel more capable. Your new energy and muscle power will encourage you to try other forms of exercise, including activities you abandoned years ago or have watched from the sidelines.

Play!

One of the best ways to work out is to play. What recreational sports did you love as a kid—swimming? bike riding? canoeing? Try them again. Now that you're fitter, you'll find them easier and more enjoyable.

Have you ever envied people who take active holidays? No reason you can't try scuba diving or snowshoeing. Think of activities you can do with your family, such as hiking or bowling. Join friends who play racquetball, tennis, or golf. One Department of Transportation Fitness Center member, a man in his mid-fifties, had been doing Quick Fit for two years when he decided to take lessons in ballroom dancing. This was something he'd always wanted to learn. Now he's out dancing every weekend.

Join a Fitness Center

Whether it's called a health club, gym, or fitness center, this is a place where you can use a wide variety of equipment and attend exercise classes. Some clubs offer additional services, such as massages or seminars on health. The social scene can be a plus, too.

Some people assume that they're too old, too fat, or too out-of-shape for a gym. That's a shame, because fitness centers aren't just for the young and hard-bodied. According to industry statistics, more than half of health club members are age thirty-five or older. If you join, chances are you won't be the heaviest or the least fit.

Another reassurance: Joining a health club doesn't have to break the bank. If your budget is tight, try your local Y or community center. Many offer superb facilities at excellent rates.

If you think you might enjoy the exercise options and camaraderie that health clubs can provide, visit nearby facilities to see what they're like. Many offer free day passes to prospective members. If the first place doesn't appeal to you, look at another—they're not all the same. Some tips on checking out a health club:

- Visit at the time of day you expect to work out. Is the club crowded? Will you have to wait in line to use the treadmill?
- Look at the equipment. Is it in good repair?
- Talk to the instructors. Are they helpful and well-informed?
- Visit the locker rooms and give them the sniff test. Is the club clean?
- Chat with members. Do they like the club?
- Ask yourself: Would I enjoy exercising here?

Take a Class

Exercise classes can be a blast, with energizing music and fun moves. They're also a great way to learn new forms of exercise, such as yoga and tai chi, because you get personal help from an instructor. Check out the offerings at your local health club, community center, Y, and adult education program. Pay attention to the descriptions: Some classes are appropriate for beginners; others are designed to challenge active young adults. If you aren't sure the level is right for you, talk to the instructor before you sign up.

EXERCISE VIDEOS

If you'd like to learn some new moves in the privacy of your own home, without having to attend a class, try an exercise video. Here are a few that are appropriate for Quick Fit veterans:

- *One Mile Walk*, by Leslie Sansone, guides you through the low-impact aerobics equivalent of a brisk one-mile walk, all done in a small area in front of your TV. Other Leslie Sansone walking videos offer similar workouts. See *http://www.lesliesansone.com*.
- *Sweatin' to the Oldies*, by Richard Simmons, provides twenty-two minutes of low-impact aerobics, performed to hits from the 1950s and 1960s. The *Sweatin' to the Oldies* series features people of all sizes. See *http://www.richardsimmons.com*.

- *Kathy Smith's March to Fitness* is slightly more challenging than the videos above, with thirty minutes of low-impact aerobic marching and dancing. See *http://www.kathysmith.com*.
- *Get Fit Fast,* a series by Denise Austin, consists of three strengthening videos that target different parts of the body: Abs; arms and shoulders; legs and buns. Each provides three workout levels, from beginning to advanced. See *http://www.deniseaustin.com*.

Some public libraries offer exercise videos. They can be rented at video shops and purchased at most bookstores. Collage Video (800-433-6769; *http://www.collagevideo.com*), which specializes in exercise tapes and DVDs, offers more than 700 titles.

EXPANDED QUICK FIT: MORE FIT, LESS QUICK

When you're ready to graduate from regular Quick Fit, you can move on to Quick Fit Plus, doing more strenuous versions of the exercises—the instructions in Chapter 6 explained how to move up. Or you can expand your workout. Which is best? Go for the version you'll do consistently.

If fifteen minutes is all you can realistically manage, do Quick Fit Plus. Your workouts won't be longer but they'll be more vigorous, which increases benefits to your health. On the other hand, you may find a demanding workout less enjoyable. In that case, Expanded Quick Fit is a better bet. You can easily increase your Quick Fit workout so that you are exercising for a total of twenty minutes, thirty minutes, or even longer. Do this gradually, so you don't overextend yourself. Here are recommendations for each part of the program:

Adding Aerobic Activity

Increasing aerobic activity piles up the benefits. If your aerobic exercise is twice as long—twenty minutes instead of ten—you'll burn double the calories. Your heart and lungs will get more of a workout, too.

If walking is your preferred aerobic activity, just take a longer walk. Similarly, you can easily increase the time you spend on Quick Steps. Either way, don't increase it by more than five minutes each week. This allows your body to accommodate easily. You can advance from ten to twenty minutes of daily aerobic activity in two weeks. And if you want to go for thirty minutes—which would meet the U.S. surgeon general's guidelines—you'll be there in a month.

It's just as effective to do your extra exercise in separate sessions. Experts used to assume that aerobic activity didn't accomplish much unless the effort was sustained for at least thirty minutes. But as we now know from numerous research studies, this isn't true (see box for one recent study). Short workouts add up, just like pocket change. And splitting up your exercise often makes it a lot easier to fit into your schedule.

DO THE MATH: 10 X 3 = 30

Researchers at the University of Ulster in Northern Ireland recruited twenty-one middle-aged men and women for a walking program. These folks were certified couch potatoes: Over the past three months they'd spent less than twenty minutes *per week* in planned physical activity.

Everyone was told to walk briskly for thirty minutes a day. But half the group did their walking all at once, while the others took three ten-minute walks daily. After six weeks they were given a vacation. Then they swapped programs.

Before and after each six-week period, they came to the lab for extensive testing. The results (which were published in *Medicine & Science in Sports & Exercise* in 2002): It didn't matter how the volunteers got their thirty minutes of exercise, in one long walk or three short ones. Everyone enjoyed the same benefits: Improved aerobic fitness, lower blood pressure, and lower cholesterol. What's more, all the participants experienced significant drops in tension and anxiety.

Pumping Up Your Strength Training

The extra exercises below—which can be completed in five or six minutes—add even more benefits to the basic Quick Fit moves. You can easily slip them into your regular workout. Or you can turn them into a separate pick-me-up exercise session for another time in the day.

Use the same dumbbells you use for the other Quick Fit

exercises. If you've moved up, you might need to dig out your starter dumbbells when you begin, since you'll be working different muscles. But you'll soon graduate to your regular pair. See pages 158–159 for guidelines on adjusting the weights.

SHOULDER CIRCLE

This simple exercise stretches your shoulder muscles as well as strengthening them, because you move your shoulders through their full range of motion. As you perform the exercise, you're activating all the muscles in your shoulders. When you strengthen the muscles around a joint, you improve the joint's stability and reduce the risk of injury. If you've suffered from aches and pains in your shoulders, don't

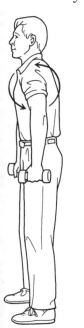
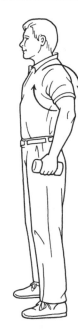

be surprised if there's a significant improvement after the muscles become stronger.

Starting Position

• Stand up tall—back straight, chest up, stomach in—with your feet flat on the floor and shoulder-width apart. There should be a slight bend in your knees, so you're comfortable and well-balanced. This is the same starting position you use for the Biceps Curls.

- Grasp the dumbbells firmly, holding one in each hand. Start with both arms at your sides, the palms parallel and facing your thighs.

The Moves

- Make forward circles with your shoulders: Lift both shoulders up and to the front. Move them down in front, then pull them back and move them up again until you've completed a circle that's as large as possible. Let your arms hang throughout the move.
- Make backward circles with your shoulders: Lift both shoulders up and to the back. Move them down in back, then pull them to the front and move them up again until you've completed a big circle. Let your arms hang.

Repetitions

- Make ten forward circles with your shoulders.
- Make ten backward circles with your shoulders.

Form Check

✔ Are you standing tall, with knees slightly bent?
✔ Are the circles as large as possible?
✔ Are you moving smoothly?

What to Watch Out For

Pay attention to your posture. Some people lean forward or back when they do this exercise. But your body should be kept straight. Also watch out for jerky movements—keep it smooth.

Customizing

Quick Fit Lite: If your regular dumbbells are too heavy, use lighter ones or do the exercise without weights at first. This will increase the flexibility and range of motion in your shoulders. Once your muscles become stronger, you can gradually add weight.

Quick Fit Plus: If ten circles in each direction is too easy, gradually increase the weight.

STANDING TRICEPS EXTENSION

The triceps muscles are in back of our upper arms. Most of us have weak triceps. That's why our arms quickly tire when we're changing an overhead lightbulb. This exercise strengthens and firms the triceps. After a few months, you'll see less jiggle in your upper arms.

Like other Quick Fit exercises, the Standing Triceps Extension delivers bonuses. Your abs get a workout, too: You'll feel them stabilize your body each time one of your arms moves back. The move also stretches your lats (the flat muscles on the side of your torso, under your arms), as well as the front of your shoulders and your upper chest.

Starting Position

- Stand up tall—back straight, chest up, stomach in—with your feet shoulder-width apart and a slight bend in your knees. This is the same position you use for the Biceps Curl.
- Grasp one dumbbell in each hand. Start with both arms at your sides, the palms parallel and facing your thighs.

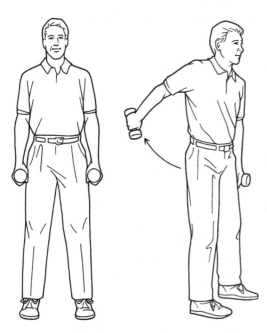

The Move

- Without bending your elbow, move your right arm straight back as far as you comfortably can.
- Return your right arm to the starting position.
- Move your left arm straight back in the same way, then return to the starting position.

Repetitions

Repeat, alternating right and left arms, until you have completed ten extensions with each arm.

Form Check

✔ Are you standing tall, with knees slightly bent?

✔ Are you facing front, without twisting?

✔ Do your arms move straight back, not out to the side?

✔ Are your elbows straight, but not locked?

What to Watch Out For

As your arm moves back, you may be tempted to lean forward or twist your body—don't! Remember that you're working your abs by holding yourself in an upright position, standing tall and facing front.

A common mistake with this exercise is to swing the weights. Move slowly and deliberately to give your muscles a safe and effective workout.

Customizing

Quick Fit Lite: If your regular dumbbells are too heavy, use lighter ones or do the exercise without weights at first. Once your muscles are stronger, you can gradually add weight.

Quick Fit Plus: If this exercise is too easy, gradually increase the weight.

FOREARM TWIST

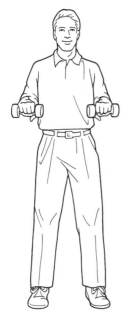

This super-simple exercise strengthens the muscles and tendons in your wrists, forearms, and biceps. If you spend a lot of time working at a keyboard, this move could help prevent repetitive strain injuries (see box on page 188).

Starting Position

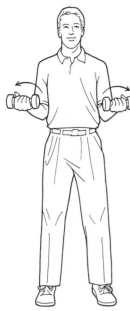

- Stand up tall—back straight, chest up, stomach in—with your feet shoulder-width apart and a slight bend in your knees. This is the same position you use for the Biceps Curl.
- Grasp one dumbbell in each hand. Both arms are at your sides, the palms parallel and facing your thighs.
- Bend your elbows, bringing both arms up just far enough so that your forearms and upper arms form a right angle. This is the starting position: Your forearms are parallel to the floor; your palms are facing each other, with the dumbbells held vertically.

The Move

- Keeping your elbows close to your body, rotate your wrists so that your thumbs move toward each other. Your palms are now facing the floor.

- Rotate your wrists so that your thumbs move away from each other. Your palms are now facing the ceiling.
- Return to the starting position, with your palms facing each other. Only your forearms should move during the exercise, rotating your wrists and your hands.

Repetitions

Repeat, rotating your wrists first toward each other and then away from each other, until you have completed ten twists in both directions.

Form Check

✔ Are you standing tall, with knees slightly bent?
✔ Are you holding your elbows close to your body?
✔ Does your forearm remain at a 90-degree angle to your upper arm throughout the move?

What to Watch Out For

As you rotate your forearms, make sure they remain perpendicular to your body rather than dropping or moving up. Stand straight and avoid leaning backward or arching your back.

Customizing

Quick Fit Lite: If your regular dumbbells are too heavy, use lighter ones or do the exercise without weights at first. Once your wrist and forearm muscles are stronger, you can gradually add weight.

Quick Fit Plus: If this exercise is too easy, gradually increase the weight.

REPETITIVE STRAIN INJURIES

- Do you often experience pain or tingling in your hands, wrists, or elbows?
- Is it difficult or painful to grip something with your hands?
- Do you find yourself massaging your hands, wrists, arms, or elbows?

If you answered Yes to any of these questions, you might have a repetitive strain injury (RSI): Damage to nerves or tendons that's caused by excessive use of your hands or arms. It's a common problem for people who use a keyboard on the job. But anyone who performs repeated hand movements—including artists, musicians, grocery cashiers, meat cutters, and sports or video game enthusiasts—is at risk. Carpal tunnel syndrome and tennis elbow are two of the best-known forms of RSIs.

Seek medical advice promptly if you experience the symptoms above. If not addressed, RSIs can cause permanent disability. Strengthening exercises help prevent the problem.

HIP BRIDGE

This move is great for the entire torso. It strengthens muscles in the back, but doesn't involve leaning backward, which would put pressure on the bones and disks in your spine. You'll work your abs, too. But there's more. Hip Bridges tone and tighten the gluteus muscles in your buttocks (called glutes). Stronger glutes improve your rear view and add power to every step you take.

You'll also feel this move in your quadriceps (or quads), the muscles in front of your thighs. Strengthening your quads supports your knee joints. If walking makes your knees ache, you may see an improvement as your quadriceps become stronger.

Note: Though the Hip Bridge is safe for most people, check with your doctor first if you have low back problems or other physical limitations.

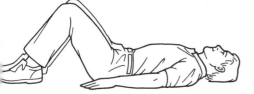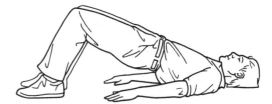

Starting Position

- Lie on your back on the floor. Your head should be on the floor; use a small pillow, if desired (see box on page 133).
- Bend your knees and place your feet flat on the floor, with your heels one to two feet away from your buttocks.

- Tilt your pelvis up slightly, so that the small of your back presses against the floor. So far, this is the same starting position you use for the Abdominal Crunches and Floor Bench Presses.
- Place your arms at your sides with your palms on the floor.

The Move

- Lift your hips six to nine inches off the floor by pushing down on your legs. Imagine your hips moving straight up toward the ceiling.
- At the top of the move, your lower back will be off the floor and your thighs will form a straight line with your abdomen. Your shoulders and head will remain flat on the floor.
- Gently lower yourself back to the starting position.

Repetitions

Repeat ten times.

Form Check

✔ When you're in the starting position, is your back flat on the floor?

✔ When you're in the "up" position, are your thighs in line with your abdomen?

What to Watch Out For

The most common mistake made with this exercise is to lift the hips higher than nine inches from the floor, which means that the abdomen and thighs are not in a straight line. This puts strain on your back.

You may find that your torso slides away from your feet with each lift. If that happens, reposition your feet between repetitions so that they're one to two feet away from your buttocks. Also, focus on lifting your hips straight up.

Customizing

Quick Fit Lite: If ten repetitions are too difficult, do five. As your torso becomes stronger, gradually work your way up to ten repetitions.

Quick Fit Plus: If ten repetitions are not sufficiently challenging, gradually work your way up to fifteen.

Stretching Your Flexibility Routine

Flexibility is essential to fitness, but it's often overlooked. As our muscles contract, they shorten. Stretching lengthens them again, restoring our range of motion. Our movements remain fluid and efficient, rather than hobbled and constrained. These two new moves address areas that often need a good stretch: The shoulders and the ankles.

CHEST AND SHOULDER STRETCH

If you spend your days hunched over a desk, this stretch will feel wonderful. It opens the chest, allowing you to breathe easier, and releases tension from the shoulders, neck, and upper back.

Starting Position

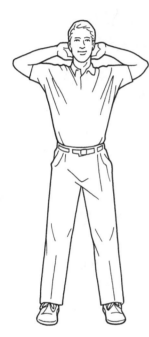

- Stand up tall—back straight, chest up, stomach in— with your feet flat on the floor and shoulder-width apart. There should be a slight bend in your knees, so you're comfortable and well balanced. This is the same position you use for the Biceps Curls.
- Put your fingertips behind your head, with your elbows out to the sides. Keep your head up straight; do not allow your hands to bend your neck forward.

The Move

- Pull your elbows back as far as you can comfortably. You will feel your shoulder blades move together.
- Hold this position to a slow count of ten.
- Relax and briefly return to the starting position.

Repetitions

Repeat twice.

Where You'll Feel the Stretch

You'll feel the stretch in your shoulders, chest, and upper back.

Form Check

✔ Are you standing with your chest up, back straight, and stomach in?
✔ Is your head up, with your chin parallel to the floor?

What to Watch Out For

Don't allow your fingers to push your head forward. The move should feel good, with your elbows back far enough for you to feel a stretch, but never out of your comfort range.

Customizing

Quick Fit Lite: If it's difficult to hold the stretch for ten seconds, maintain it for five seconds. Gradually work your way up to ten seconds.

Quick Fit Plus: Work toward expanding your range of motion, but don't pull your elbows back so far that the stretch becomes uncomfortable.

TOE CIRCLE

Strong, flexible ankles help maintain our balance, even when we're walking on uneven surfaces. This move tones and stretches the ankles, reducing the risk of sprains or falls. And because the exercise is done with your legs extended, it also strengthens your quadriceps, the muscles on top of your thighs. Stronger quads stabilize your knee joints. That's quite a payoff for a one-minute exercise! You can do this simple move any time you're stuck in a chair and want to improve circulation in your legs.

Starting Position

- Sit tall in a sturdy chair, with your feet flat on the floor.
- If the chair has arms, grasp them gently. Otherwise, gently grasp the seat.

The Moves

- Extend your right leg straight out, leaving a slight bend in your knee so that the joint is not locked.
- Draw big circles in the air by turning your ankle to the right (clockwise) and pointing your toe. Your leg should remain motionless, except for your ankle.

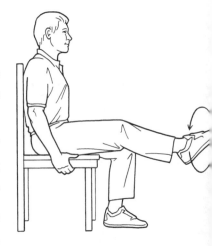

- Return to the starting position.
- Extend your left leg straight out, leaving a slight bend in your knee.
- Point your left toe forward, then draw big circles in the air by bending and turning your ankle to the right (clockwise). Your leg should remain motionless, except for your ankle.
- Return to the starting position.
- Lift your right leg as before, but this time bend your ankle so your right toe draws circles to the left (counterclockwise).
- Return to the starting position.
- Lift your left leg as before, but this time bend your ankle so your left toe draws circles to the left (counterclockwise).

Repetitions

- Draw ten clockwise circles with your right toe.
- Draw ten clockwise circles with your left toe.
- Draw ten counterclockwise circles with your right toe.
- Draw ten counterclockwise circles with your left toe.

Where You'll Feel the Stretch

You'll feel the stretch in your foot and ankle. You'll also feel tightening in your thigh as your quadriceps contract to hold your leg up.

Form Check

✔ Is there a slight bend in your knee, so that the joint doesn't lock?

✔ Is your leg extended and steady throughout the move?

What to Watch Out For

The most common problem with this exercise is movement in the leg. Make sure you hold your leg steady and that only your ankle moves.

Customizing

Quick Fit Lite: If it's too difficult to draw ten circles in each direction with each leg, start with five and work your way up.

Quick Fit Plus: If it's very easy to draw ten circles, move a little faster and draw up to fifteen circles in each direction with each leg.

Putting It All Together

You've learned the new moves. Now, decide how you'd like to incorporate them into your day.

You can easily increase your Quick Fit workout to twenty minutes, thirty minutes, or even longer. See the box for a summary of the Expanded Quick Fit workout. Add as many of the optional moves as you wish—but be sure to do all the required exercises.

Feel free to improvise with the new exercises. For example, you might decide to add the optional strengthening moves to your usual Quick Fit workout, and to do the two new stretches during the day when you need a break. Or you might prefer to continue with your regular Quick Fit workout, but to add the new exercises by doing a second workout during the day. If so, end that session with a Sit and Reach stretch.

Quick Fit has shown you how much fifteen minutes of daily exercise can accomplish. By adding a little more—and doing it consistently—you can increase the benefits.

I suggest you build upon Quick Fit rather than start a completely new routine. This will give you a solid foundation, one that you know is effective. When you make it a personal goal to do Quick Fit every day—even on those days when you can't do more—you'll always have the satisfaction of success.

RICK BRADLEY'S EXPANDED QUICK FIT WORKOUT

PART 1: AEROBIC EXERCISE (10 OR MORE MINUTES)

OPTION 1: Walk on the treadmill at three miles per hour

OPTION 2: Walk outdoors at three miles per hour

OPTION 3: Quick Steps

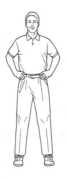

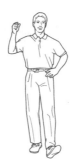

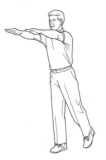

- MARCH
  (one minute)

- FRONT HEEL
  TOUCH
  (one minute)
- MARCH
  (one minute)

- BACK TOE TOUCH
  (one minute)
- MARCH
  (one minute)

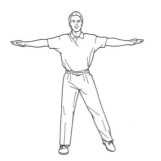

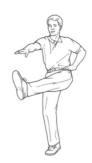

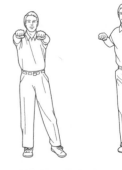

- SIDE TOUCH (one minute)
- MARCH (one minute)

- FRONT KICK
  (one minute)
- MARCH
  (one minute)

- HAMSTRING CURL
  (one minute)

198   from *Quick Fit: The Complete 15-Minute No-Sweat Workout*
by Richard Bradley III, with Sarah Wernick (Atria Books, 2004)

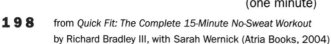

PART 2: ABDOMINAL STRENGTHENING EXERCISE (1 MINUTE)

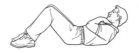

- ABDOMINAL CRUNCH (two sets of ten repetitions)

PART 3: UPPER BODY AND MIDSECTION STRENGTHENING EXERCISES (3 MINUTES)

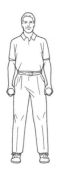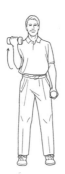

- BICEPS CURL (ten repetitions with each arm)

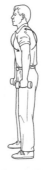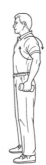

- SHOULDER CIRCLE (ten repetitions in each direction—optional)

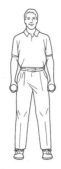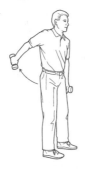

- STANDING TRICEPS EXTENSION (ten repetitions with each arm—optional)

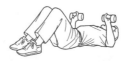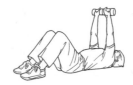

- FLOOR BENCH PRESS (ten repetitions)

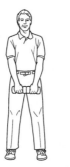
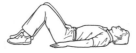
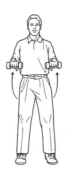
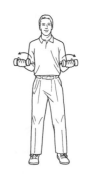
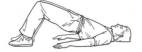

- STANDING ROW
  (ten repetitions)

- FOREARM TWIST
  (ten repetitions—optional)

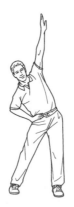

- HIP BRIDGE (ten repetitions—optional)

PART 4: STRETCHES

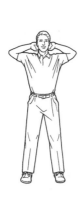
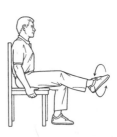
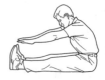

- TOE CIRCLE (ten circles to left and
  to right with each leg—optional)

- CHEST AND
  SHOULDER
  STRETCH (two ten
  second stretches—
  optional)

- SIDE BEND
  (thirty seconds
  or ten bends
  to each side)

- SIT AND REACH
  (thirty seconds)

http://www.ricksquickfit.com

chapter nine

QUESTIONS AND ANSWERS

If you were attending one of my seminars, I'd call for questions at this point. Is your hand up? I hope you'll find the answers you need in this chapter. If not, try the index.

You may find it helpful to reread the book after you've been doing Quick Fit for a while. You'll have a different perspective then, and you'll probably pick up points you missed the first time around.

GETTING STARTED

Q: I haven't begun Quick Fit, because I plan to walk outdoors and it's been too cold. Does it pay to do the other exercises even if I can't do the walk?

A: Definitely start the other exercises! With physical activity, doing something is always better than doing nothing. However, this experience shows that you need a backup plan for bad weather. Quick Steps—marching in place with variations—is perfect for those occasions (see pages 110–117). I hope you will try it.

Q: I've just learned that I'm pregnant. Can I start Quick Fit?

A: Congratulations—and here's to a healthy pregnancy and baby. Quick Fit is safe for nearly everyone, including most mothers-to-be. But talk to your doctor, just to be sure you can do the workout without modifications.

The American College of Obstetricians and Gynecologists encourages pregnant women to exercise regularly, unless there's a specific medical reason not to. In addition to all the other health benefits of exercise, fitness may make childbirth a little easier.

Q: How soon after my baby is born can I begin Quick Fit?

A: Exercise is great for new moms! Physical activity can help you get back in shape. A workout boosts your energy just when you need it most. And exercise helps counter postpartum depression.

Your doctor probably will encourage you to walk before you leave the hospital, even if you've had a cesarean. Short walks, at a comfortable pace, will help your body recover and prepare you for more vigorous exercise. However, your joints remain loose because of the hormonal changes of pregnancy. So don't begin or resume Quick Fit's strengthening exercises and stretches until you've consulted your doctor at your post-partum checkup.

Q: My children—ages five, eight, and twelve—have been asking if they can do Quick Fit with me. Is this program okay for kids?

A: What a great example you're setting for your children! And you can see that it's working, because they want to join you.

If your children have medical clearance to participate in physical education at school or child care, then it's safe for them to do Quick Fit's aerobic exercise and stretches. Youngsters should be supervised if they're using a treadmill. And if your family does Quick Steps together, make sure you all have enough room to move without bumping into one another.

The strengthening exercises are also safe for most children—but the American Academy of Pediatrics (AAP) advises that youngsters receive clearance from a pediatrician before beginning a strength training program. When you talk to your children's doctor, explain that Quick Fit uses light weights, and ask about any limits that you should place upon the weights they lift.

AAP recommends that children first learn strengthening exercises without weights. When they've mastered the proper form, they can gradually add weight, following the pediatrician's recommendations. Teach them to treat the weights with respect, always handling them carefully and storing them safely when they're not in use. Most important:

Encourage your children to see themselves as a team, not as competitors.

GENERAL QUESTIONS ABOUT QUICK FIT

Q: I'm planning to do Quick Fit during my lunch hour. Should I exercise before or after I eat?

A: Either way is fine, so go by your own preference. You may have heard warnings against strenuous activity just after a meal. But moderate-intensity exercise like Quick Fit usually doesn't interfere with digestion. See if you feel comfortable doing brisk walking or abdominal crunches after you eat. If not, schedule your workout first. Also consider convenience. If you're exercising at a fitness center, the treadmills may be less busy at the end of lunch hour than at the beginning.

Q: If I do Quick Fit just before I go to bed, will it interfere with my sleep?

A: Probably not. But Quick Fit does increase your metabolism a little bit. If you find that falling asleep is a problem after a nighttime workout, figure out another way to fit the program into your day.

Q: I work shifts and my schedule varies. Can I do Quick Fit at different times on different days?

A: Yes—it doesn't matter when you do it, so long as you get it done. But you'll find it easier to remain consistent if you tie Quick Fit to the predictable parts of your schedule. For example, you could do it right after you wake up, whenever that happens to be. You could also do it just before or after a meal.

Q: I have a bad back and I know I need to exercise. However, it's very difficult for me to get down on the floor, and even harder to get up again. Any suggestions, other than doing the exercise on a bed?

A: Here's a technique that will help you get down on the floor if you suffer from back pain or minor balance problems. (Note: This method doesn't work for everyone. For example, it's not appropriate unless you're able to kneel. If you have physical limitations, ask a physical therapist or personal trainer for customized suggestions.)

You'll need a sturdy chair with a wide seat and no armrests. Don't use a folding chair or one with wheels. For stability, a wooden chair is better than one with a cushioned seat.

- Position the chair just next to your workout space, with its back against a wall so it won't slide.
- Face the chair. Place both hands flat on the chair seat, about six inches apart, with your fingers pointing toward the back of the chair. Lean on the chair with both hands.
- Using your hands for support and balance, get down on one knee. When that knee is on the ground, get down on the other knee. You're now kneeling on both knees in front

of the chair, with your hands supporting part of your weight.

- Slide your right hand to the middle of the chair. Place your left hand on the floor about twelve inches to the left of the chair. (Switch hands if that would be easier for you.)
- Using your hands for support, roll onto your left hip. (If you've switched hands, roll onto your right hip.)
- Straighten out your legs and roll onto your rear end. You are now sitting on the floor.

After you've finished your floor exercises, get up by reversing the process:

- Roll onto one hip, positioning yourself so that you're facing the chair and about twelve inches away from it.
- Using your hands for support, roll onto your knees, so you're kneeling on both knees in front of the chair.
- Put both hands flat on the chair seat, about six inches apart, with fingers pointing to the back of the chair.
- Using your hands for support, lift one knee and put your foot flat on the floor. Rise, pushing up with that leg and with your hands.

USING A BED FOR QUICK FIT

My mother, who's eighty-one years old, recently started Quick Fit. Getting down and up from the floor is more than she can manage. So she does the floor exercises on her bed.

After she finishes her Abdominal Crunches, she brings the dumbbells to the bed. She stands facing the end of the bed and does the Biceps Curls. Then she turns around, sits on the bed, and lies down to do the Floor Bench Presses. She stands up again for the Standing Row. All this time, the bed serves as a convenient "rack" for the dumbbells. She puts them away and finishes her workout with the two stretches.

AEROBIC ACTIVITY

Q: I have severe osteoarthritis in my knees and can't stand on my feet for ten minutes. Walking and Quick Steps are impossible for me. Is there any way I can do Quick Fit?

A: Yes! And I think you will benefit greatly from physical activity. Please talk to your doctor about this program. Ask if any of the following options are appropriate for you:

- Quick Steps in a chair: Sit on a sturdy chair with no arms and begin to march. You can do the variations in which your legs move to the front or side: Front Heel Touch (pages 112–113), Side Touch (pages 114–115), and Front Kick (pages 115–116). If you move vigorously, chair exercise can be surprisingly strenuous.
- Cycling or stationary cycling: The muscles in your lower body will get a workout, and so will your heart and lungs.

- Cycling with an upper body ergometer: This device— available at some fitness centers—looks like a stationary bicycle, but it's powered by your arms rather than your legs.
- Rowing or rowing machine: Rowing works the large muscles in your arms and legs, and it's also a good aerobic workout.
- Swimming or water aerobics: The water makes you nearly weightless and also provides resistance, so you can get a good workout without stress to your knees.

As with any new exercise, obtain instructions before trying unfamiliar equipment, such as an upper body ergometer or rowing machine. Start at a low intensity and increase gradually. For example, if you're using a stationary cycle, set it to a light resistance level at first and pedal at a speed that's comfortable for you. These precautions are especially important if physical limitations make you vulnerable to injury.

Q: I'd like to buy a treadmill, but the motorized versions are so expensive. What about nonmotorized treadmills?

A: I don't recommend nonmotorized treadmills. All of them require you to walk on an incline of at least 3 percent. Walking uphill puts more of a strain on your body than walking on a level surface. With a nonmotorized treadmill, your legs are not only walking but also pushing the belt. That makes the movement more difficult and less natural.

You can find treadmill reviews in back issues of *Runner's World* and *Consumer Reports,* which may be available at your library. Try before you buy: Some treadmills feel more comfortable than others when you walk on them.

Remember, you don't need a treadmill to do Quick Fit. Walking is free. And so is Quick Steps if you prefer to exercise indoors.

Q: I'm ready to increase the intensity of my aerobic activity. Any reason I can't jog or run instead of walk?

A: Unless your body is used to running—as mine is—I recommend walking for people who are doing Quick Fit. When you walk, at least one foot is on the ground at all times. But when you run or jog, both feet are in the air simultaneously, so your body lands with much more impact. That increases the risk of muscle strain, damage to joints, and other injury— especially for people whose bodies aren't accustomed to strenuous exercise. Why take chances when brisk walking gives you an excellent aerobic workout?

ABDOMINAL EXERCISE

Q: I have one of those C-shaped ab gizmos that supports my head as I work my abs. Can I use that when I do the Abdominal Crunches?

A: Yes, you can use your ab machine for Quick Fit. But it's better to do the exercise without it, because you give your neck muscles a workout, too. (See box about neck support on page 125.)

Q: What about those sliding ab machines—are they helpful?

A: I emphatically recommend against using them. With these machines, you kneel and grab onto handles that move forward on the floor or along a track. Your knees remain in one spot while your upper body stretches forward, elongating your abdominal muscles. But at the same time, those muscles must contract to prevent your body from collapsing onto the floor. There's a real risk of muscular strain and rips, as well as an abdominal hernia (a condition in which the intestines protrude through a tear in the abdominal muscles).

STRENGTHENING EXERCISES

Q: I'd like to become stronger, but I'm a woman and don't want to develop big muscles. Will Quick Fit make my arms look bulky?

A: We're all bound to develop muscles if we exercise, but that doesn't mean we get muscle-bound. Bodybuilders develop their bulky muscles with heavy weights and long workouts. Your Quick Fit strengthening exercises use light weights and take just four minutes a day. They will make your muscles firmer and more toned but won't turn you into the Incredible Hulk.

Q: Instead of buying weights, can I use cans or milk jugs filled with sand or water?

A: It's safe to use cans, provided you can hold them securely. In practice, that limits you to one-pound cans. But you won't get the same strengthening benefit that you'd get from heavier weights.

Milk jugs were not designed for strength training, and I don't recommend them. Their handles are small and may become uncomfortable during a workout. If you're making a commitment to follow the Quick Fit program, I suggest you invest in a pair of inexpensive dumbbells.

Q: Can I use one of those stretchy exercise tubes instead of dumbbells?

A: Exercise tubes give you a good workout. They're great for travel, because they're so light and compact. But over time they wear out, and they can tear or lose their elasticity. So I don't recommend them for everyday use. If you plan to buy some for travel, select the kind with handles. They're easier on your wrists than the bands that you must wrap around your hands to grip.

Q: Can I do Quick Fit with the strength training machines at the gym?

A: Dumbbells are better for Quick Fit—and they're also available at the gym. Most strength training machines don't have weight settings that are light enough for this program. Also, the numbering systems vary from brand to brand, so it's difficult to be consistent if you use different machines. But any five-pound dumbbell weighs five pounds.

Q: Don't I have to rest for a day after doing exercises with weights?

A: Not if you're doing Quick Fit. One approach to strengthening exercise involves lifting heavy weights until your muscles are exhausted. That sounds painful—and it often is. The exertion actually creates tiny tears in your muscle fibers. Your body repairs the tears; in the process, you become stronger. But you may also feel sore.

People who lift heavy weights must rest their muscles for at least a day between workouts, to allow time for these repairs. But Quick Fit uses light weights, so it's perfectly safe to perform these strengthening exercises every day. If you experience muscle soreness, that's a signal that your weights are too heavy, so switch to lighter weights.

Q: I've read that you get better results with strength training if you do the moves very slowly. Should I do it that way?

A: Not unless you're looking for tedium and discomfort. With super-slow weight lifting (sometimes called Slo-Mo), you take fourteen to twenty seconds for each repetition, rather than the conventional three to eight seconds. Most people find slow lifting extremely boring—and the workout takes longer. Also, you can expect muscle soreness if you do the Quick Fit program this way. That's because your muscles get no help from momentum or gravity when you move slowly, so they have to work harder. For all these reasons, I don't recommend it.

STRETCHING

Q: When I do the Side Bends, I hear popping noises in my shoulders. Should I stop doing them?

A: Noisy shoulder and knee joints are a common phenomenon. As long as there's no pain, chances are there's no problem. But if you experience any discomfort along with the popping, have the joint checked by a doctor.

Q: I spend long hours in my car and find that the Side Bends and Sit and Reach stretches relieve stiffness in my back and shoulders. Can I do them more often than once a day?

A: So long as you don't stretch past the comfort point, you can stretch as often as you like! I recommend frequent quick stretching breaks throughout the day.

RICK'S FITNESS ROUTINE

Q: Rick, do you do Quick Fit?

A: Yes, I occasionally do Quick Fit Plus, with a jog instead of a walk and with heavier weights. But that's only if there's no time for my usual forty-five-minute exercise routine.

Remember, fitness is my profession and my passion. And besides, my body needs to move.

Normally, I start by running a couple of miles over a route in my neighborhood. I like to run first thing in the morning, because it gets me pumped for the day. The run takes about twenty minutes. When I come back, I do 100 sit-ups, 60 push-ups, and 60 pull-ups on a chinning bar that I've installed in my basement. Is this part fun? Not exactly, but neither is brushing and flossing. I listen to the morning news and I'm done by the time they give the weather report. Then I finish up with five minutes of stretching, and head for the shower.

I've been following this routine since I graduated from high school. I'm past fifty now, and I've never felt better in my life. I can still fit into the suit I wore to my college graduation, and when I play tennis with my son, Ryan—who was on his college team—he has to work hard to win. Fitness has been good to me. Even if you never do as much exercise as I do, it will be good to you, too.

TROUBLESHOOTING

Q: I keep meaning to start Quick Fit, but it's not happening! Any suggestions?

A: The toughest part of an exercise program is taking the first step. Once you're past that, the exercises themselves will be a cinch.

Two dozen volunteers offered to test the program for this book. We gave them the instructions. A week later, we sent everyone a note asking "How's it going?" Several people confessed that they hadn't yet started—but they promised to begin the next day. And guess what: They did! That simple reminder did the trick.

Here are a few ideas for using reminders to give yourself an extra push:

- Set a reasonable deadline for starting, and note it on your calendar.
- Write yourself a letter listing all the reasons you want to get fit—and mail it.
- Tape the letter to your bathroom mirror so you see it every day.
- Ask a friend to call in a week to ask, "Are you doing Quick Fit?"
- Order the weights (see page 93 for telephone and internet sources), so they'll be available when you're ready.
- Set up your workout area, and make it as inviting as possible.
- Leave this book on your kitchen table or in some other visible spot, with a place marker on page 101. That's where you'll find Quick Start, which tells you how to begin Quick Fit before you've read the whole book. Remember, this program takes just fifteen minutes; Quick Start lets you begin with ten, adding one exercise each day for a week.

Q: I missed my Quick Fit workout today. Should I do it twice tomorrow to make up?

A: No—you could develop muscle soreness if you do twice as much as your body expects. Also, it would be harder to find time for a double workout, which might cause you to skip a second day.

An occasional missed workout isn't a problem. But if this is happening more than once or twice a week, consider that a red flag. Read pages 164–165 for suggestions on how to get back on track.

Q: I've been doing Quick Fit and I'm starting to feel stiff and achy. What should I do now?

A: Sometimes people who have been very sedentary develop aches and pains after they start Quick Fit. Most often, the problem is temporary; usually it disappears in a week or even in a few days.

Here are questions to consider:

- Is the problem associated with walking—in other words, do you have discomfort in your feet, legs, hips, knees, or lower back? If so, check your shoes. Proper footwear can make a big difference. See pages 95–100 for recommendations.
- Are you overdoing it? Sometimes people are so enthusiastic about Quick Fit that they advance too rapidly. They feel fine during their workouts, but a day or two later, they develop muscle soreness. If you started out with Quick Fit

Plus, try doing regular Quick Fit for a while. If you had been very sedentary and began with regular Quick Fit, try Quick Fit Lite. Follow the directions in Chapter 6 for gradually increasing the intensity of your workouts.

- Are you doing all the exercises in proper form? Reread the instructions. Even better, ask a friend to read them aloud and watch you perform the moves.

- Are your weights too heavy? You may be accustomed to strength training programs that use heavy weights and involve only two or three workouts a week. But because you're doing Quick Fit every day, you must use lighter weights.

FOR MORE INFORMATION

If you'd like more information on fitness and health, or if you're interested in going beyond Quick Fit, have a look at the following books:

- *LifeFit: An Effective Exercise Program for Optimal Health and a Longer Life*, by Ralph S. Paffenbarger Jr., M.D. and Eric Olsen (Human Kinetics, 1996). Dr. Paffenbarger founded the College Alumni Health Study described in Chapter 2. His book discusses the health benefits of exercise and offers a detailed fitness plan based on his research.

- *The Spark: The Revolutionary 3-Week Fitness Plan That*

Changes Everything You Know About Exercise, Weight Control, and Health, by Glenn A. Gaesser, Ph.D., and Karla Dougherty (Simon & Schuster, 2001). Dr. Gaesser's research at the University of Virginia showed that ten-minute periods of exercise (he calls them "sparks") can add up to a regimen that's highly effective for fitness and weight loss. The book includes a three-week exercise and diet plan.

- *The Canyon Ranch Guide to Living Younger Longer: A Complete Program for Optimal Health for Body, Mind, and Spirit*, by the staff of Canyon Ranch with Len Sherman (Simon & Schuster, 2001). This beautiful book, from one of the world's leading health resorts, explains how to make healthy living a joy.

- *The Anytime, Anywhere Exercise Book*, by Joan Price with Lawrence Kassman, M.D. (Adams Media, 2003). This book offers 300-plus quick and easy moves—some requiring just one or two minutes—that add physical activity to your day, whether you're at home, in the office, or on the road.

- *Strong Women Stay Young*, by Miriam Nelson, Ph.D., with Sarah Wernick (revised edition, Bantam, 2000). The simple, health-focused strength training program in this book is appropriate for men as well as women. By the same authors are *Strong Women Stay Slim* (Bantam, 1999), about healthy weight loss, and *Strong Women, Strong Bones* (Perigee, 2001), about preventing and treating osteoporosis. *Strong Women and Men Beat Arthritis* (Putnam, 2002), by Dr. Nelson, Ronenn Roubenoff, M.D., and Kristin Baker, Ph.D., with Lawrence Lindner, contains extensive information on arthritis, with an exercise program designed specifically to relieve stiffness and pain.

- *The Complete Fit or Fat Book: The New Fit or Fat/The Fit-Or-Fat Woman/The Fit-Or-Fat Target Diet/Fit-Or-Fat Target Recipes*, by Covert Bailey and Lea Bishop (Galahad Books, 2001). Covert Bailey has updated his popular book, *Fit or Fat*, and added diet information and recipes—all in one volume.
- *Stretching*, by Bob Anderson (Shelter Publications, 2000). In this revision of the classic book on the subject, you'll find basic stretching instructions, as well as specialty stretches for particular sports, times of day, and problem areas of the body.

CONSISTENCY IS THE NAME OF THE GAME

People who aren't familiar with my exercise routine some-times ask me how I stay so fit. I tell them: "I just do a lit-tle bit every day." In truth, my consistency is more important than the details of my workout.

Consistency helps us succeed in everything we do, whether it's school, work, or personal relationships. Of course, other things help, too. But with fitness, consistency is the name of the game. If you do your workout every day, you will succeed. Guaranteed.

Quick Fit is designed to make consistency as easy as pos-sible. Many people at the Department of Transportation have been doing this program ever since I introduced it in 1999—and they say they plan to stick with Quick Fit (or even more ambitious exercise regimens) forever. If they can do it, so can you.

TAKE THE PLEDGE

You've read all the way to the end of this book, so I know that becoming physically fit is important to you. I hope you're excited about Quick Fit. The time to begin the program is right now, while you're feeling strongly motivated.

Remember that pledge I told you about in Chapter 4? I'd like you to raise your right hand and say the words:

I promise to do the Quick Fit program every day.

You can take the pledge in front of your spouse, your kids, a close friend, or your boss. Or you can just read the words silently, and know that you really mean them. One way or another, make that commitment. And then get started.

WHAT TO EXPECT IN THE FIRST FOUR MONTHS

It takes about four months to see real results with Quick Fit. You'll experience plenty of improvements before then. In fact, you'll feel great right after you've completed your first workout.

Of course, everyone is different. But here's a month-by-month guide to what you can expect—and the challenges you may face—as you begin to exercise consistently:

Month 1

The most exciting day (and the toughest) of any exercise program is Day 1. You're filled with enthusiasm. The moves aren't yet familiar, so you might have to interrupt yourself to read the instructions. But when you've finished Quick Fit for the first time, you'll be delighted. Your next workout will go more smoothly. And because the program is so simple, you'll master it in just a few days.

After three days of activity, your muscles and cardiovascular system begin to acclimate themselves to exercise. After three to four weeks, if you remain consistent, your body will actually expect to move every day. That's the start of a healthy lifetime habit.

I definitely feel an immediate result after exercise. I'm mentally stimulated and more alert. I feel my body switched on.
　　　　　　—ANTHONY

Month 2

During the first month, your task was to learn the exercises. Now you're into a routine, and the challenge is to continue it consistently.

By the second month, you should see some changes. Your workouts are becoming a little easier. You may also notice improvements in your daily life, especially if you weren't active before starting Quick Fit.

At work, there's a soda machine down three flights of stairs. I had been getting winded coming back from the soda machine. The second month after I started Quick Fit, I noticed that I could take the stairs with ease.

—CLARE

Month 3

You're a Quick Fit veteran by now. Do you realize that if you've walked half a mile every day since you started, you've already completed the equivalent of a marathon? Wow!

At this point, the program is comfortable and familiar; you've established an exercise habit. This month's challenge is to keep your workouts fresh. Add some variety (see pages 160–161 for suggestions). Consider graduating to Quick Fit Plus, if you haven't already. And if you began with Quick Fit Lite, see if you can move up to the regular program.

My clothes are fitting better. Some things had

been snug, but now they're not. I noticed this after the second month.

—ANNE

Month 4

If you've done Quick Fit consistently for four months, this program is now part of your lifestyle. I hope you're enjoying the increased vitality that physical activity brings. You're feeling better and your friends are probably telling you that you look better, too. Congratulations!

You can keep doing Quick Fit every day. But you might also consider some of the options in Chapter 8 for adding even more physical activity to your life.

I like to walk outdoors at night. I walk in snow and rain. But if it's really terrible weather, what gets me out of the house is telling myself that I'm doing it for just ten minutes. Then, by the time I've done five minutes, I'm warmed up and it isn't so bad. I rarely do just the ten minutes.

—CHUCK

A LIFETIME OF FITNESS

A friend of mine says, "I exercise because I want to die young—at a very old age." What he means is that he wants to live for many years, remaining energetic, strong, and flexible to the very end. In other words: Youthful. Isn't that what all of us wish for ourselves? Exercising consistently can make it happen.

You've used Quick Fit to begin a habit of daily physical activity. Whether you continue with Quick Fit, or make it the bridge to an active lifestyle, may it be the foundation for a stronger, healthier, and happier You.

God bless—

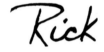

INDEX

INDEX

arthritis, 62
Austin, Denise, 178

B

back:
   lower, problems with, 189, 205–6
   pain in, 99
   strengthening, 126
   stretching, 140
back toe touch, 113–14
balance:
   problems with, 119, 205
   on treadmill, 92
ballistic stretching, 137
ballroom dancing, 175
bed, floor exercises on, 119, 206–7
biceps, strengthening, 126, 128, 186
biceps curl, 102, 128–30
biochemical changes, from exercise, 27
blisters, 97
blood circulation, 26, 28–29, 55
blood pressure, 30–31, 34, 127, 151
blood sugar, 32–33, 34
body shape:
   bulky muscles, 210
   trimmer, 150, 169
body strength, increasing, 149
bones, effects of exercise on, 27, 62
boredom, avoiding, 52–53, 212
bouncing, dangers of, 137
Bradley, Richard R. III:
   background of, 4–6, 7–8
   fitness routine of, 213–14
brain, effects of exercise on, 27
brain chemicals, 36
Brannock Device, 97
breathing, 32
   difficulty in, 106
   song test, 108
   in strengthening exercises, 127–28

buttocks muscles:
   glutes, 189
   strengthening, 189
   stretching, 140

C

calf muscles, stretching, 140
calories, burning, 25, 56, 152, 168, 179
cancer, 31–32, 34
cans, lifting, 211
cardiovascular conditions, 61
carpal tunnel syndrome, 188
catching up, 165, 216
caution, 106
celebrations, 165–66
central nervous system, effects of
   exercise on, 27
chair:
   lowering to the floor with aid of,
     205–6
   Quick Steps in, 207
chest:
   pecs, 131
   strengthening, 126, 131, 184
   tightness or pain in, 106
chest and shoulder stretch, 192–93
childbirth, and exercise, 202–3
children:
   medical clearance for, 203
   physical activity for, 78
   Quick Fit for, 203–4
   strength training for, 203
   teamwork vs. competition for, 204
   and treadmill safety, 91, 203
cholesterol, 29, 34, 151
chores, active, 172
classes, exercise, 176, 177
claudication, 29
clock with second hand, 90
clothes, 94–95

INDEX